The AOTA Practice Guidelines Series

Occupational Therapy Practice Guidelines *for*

Individuals With Work-Related Injuries and Illnesses

Vicki Kaskutas, OTD, MHS, OT/L
Instructor in Occupational Therapy and Medicine
Washington University School of Medicine

Jeff Snodgrass, PhD, MPH, OTR/L, CWCE
Program Director and Associate Professor
Occupational Therapy Program
Milligan College
Part-Time Faculty
School of Health Sciences, College of Health Sciences
Walden University

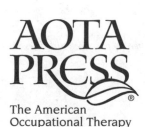

AOTA PRESS
The American
Occupational Therapy
Association, Inc.

AOTA Centennial Vision

We envision that occupational therapy is a powerful, widely recognized, science-driven, and evidence-based profession with a globally connected and diverse workforce meeting society's occupational needs.

Mission Statement

The American Occupational Therapy Association advances the quality, availability, use, and support of occupational therapy through standard-setting, advocacy, education, and research on behalf of its members and the public.

AOTA Staff

Frederick P. Somers, *Executive Director*
Christopher M. Bluhm, *Chief Operating Officer*

Chris Davis, *Director, AOTA Press*
Ashley Hofmann, *Production Editor*
Victoria Davis, *Editorial Assistant*

Beth Ledford, *Director, Marketing and Member Communications*
Emily Harlow, *Technology Marketing Specialist*
Jennifer Folden, *Marketing Specialist*

American Occupational Therapy Association, Inc.
4720 Montgomery Lane
PO Box 31220
Bethesda, MD 20814
Phone: 301-652-AOTA (2682)
TDD: 800-377-8555
Fax: 301-652-7711
www.aota.org

To order: 1-877-404-AOTA or store.aota.org

Disclaimers

This publication is designed to provided accurate and authoritative information in regard to the subject matter covered. It is sold or distributed with the understanding that the publisher is not engaged in rendering legal, accounting, or other professional service. If legal advice or other expert assistance is required, the services of a competent professional person should be sought.
—*From the Declaration of Principles jointly adopted by the American Bar Association and a Committee of Publishers and Associations*

It is the objective of the American Occupational Therapy Association to be a forum for free expression and interchange of ideas. The opinions expressed by the contributors to this work are their own and not necessarily those of the American Occupational Therapy Association.

ISBN 10: 1-56900-260-6
ISBN 13: 978-1-56900-260-5
Library of Congress Control Number: 2009925470

Cover Design by Sarah Ely and Michael Melletz
Composition by Maryland Composition, White Plains, MD
Printed by Automated Graphic Services, White Plains, MD

Reference: Kaskutas, V., & Snodgrass, J. (2009). *Occupational therapy practice guidelines for individuals with work-related injuries and illnesses.* Bethesda, MD: AOTA Press.

Contents

Appendixes

References

Figures and Tables Used in This Publication

■ ■ ■

Acknowledgments

Authors
Vicki Kaskutas, OTD, MHS, OT/L
Instructor in Occupational Therapy and Medicine
Washington University School of Medicine,
    St. Louis, MO

Jeff Snodgrass, PhD, MPH, OTR/L, CWCE
Program Director and Associate Professor
Occupational Therapy Program, Milligan College,
    Milligan College, TN
Part-Time Faculty
School of Health Sciences, College of Health
    Sciences
Walden University, Minneapolis, MN

Series Editor
Deborah Lieberman, MHSA, OTR/L, FAOTA
Program Director, Evidence-Based Practice
Staff Liaison to the Commission on Practice
American Occupational Therapy Association
Bethesda, MD

**The authors would like to acknowledge the
following individuals for their contributions to
the evidence-based literature review:**
Debbie Amini, MEd, OTR/L, CHT
Marian Arbesman, PhD, OTR/L
Paula Bohr, PhD, OTR/L, FAOTA
Jeff Snodgrass, PhD, MPH, OTR/L, CWCE
Rebecca von der Heyde, MS, OTR/L, CHT

Lynn Attaway, Stephanie Jones, Courtney McCray,
    Misty Smith, and Nicolas Tudor, who were gradu-
    ate students at Milligan College at the time of this
    work.

**The authors would like to acknowledge and
thank the following individuals for their
participation in the content review and
development of this publication:**
Debbie Amini, MEd, OTR/L, CHT
Marian Arbesman, PhD, OTR/L
Paula Bohr, PhD, OTR/L, FAOTA
Donna Colaianni, MS, OTR/L, CHT
Michael J. Gerg, MS, OTR/L, CHT, CEES, CWCE
Kathy Maltchev, OTR/L
Sheri Montgomery, OTR/L, FAOTA
Colette Nagami, OTR/L
V. Judith Thomas, MGA
Rebecca von der Heyde, MS, OTR/L, CHT
Chuck Willmarth.

**The authors thank the following individuals for
their participation in the development of the case
studies and recommendation tables included in
this publication:**
Debbie Amini, MEd, OTR/L, CHT
Paula Bohr, PhD, OTR/L, FAOTA
Jeff Snodgrass, PhD, MPH, OTR/L, CWCE
Rebecca von der Heyde, MS, OTR/L, CHT.

■ ■ ■

Introduction

Purpose and Use of This Publication

Practice guidelines have been widely developed in response to the health care reform movement in the United States. Such guidelines can be a useful tool for improving the quality of health care, enhancing consumer satisfaction, promoting appropriate use of services, and reducing costs. The American Occupational Therapy Association (AOTA), which represents the professional interests of 140,000 occupational therapists, occupational therapy assistants, and students of occupational therapy, is committed to providing information to support decision making that promotes a high-quality health care system that is affordable and accessible to all.

Using information from an evidence-based literature review, expert opinion, and key concepts from the *Occupational Therapy Practice Framework: Domain and Process* (AOTA, 2008b), this guideline provides an overview of the occupational therapy process for assessment and treatment of individuals with work-related injuries and/or illnesses that were sustained on the job. It defines the occupational therapy domain, process, and intervention that occur within the boundaries of acceptable practice. This guideline does not discuss all possible methods of care, and although it does recommend some specific methods of care, the occupational therapist makes the ultimate judgment regarding the appropriateness of a given procedure in light of a person's specific circumstances and needs.

It is the intention of AOTA, through this publication, to help occupational therapists and occupational therapy assistants, as well as the individuals who manage, reimburse, or set policy regarding occupational therapy services, understand the contribution of occupational therapy in treating individuals with work-related injuries and illnesses covered by state or federal workers' compensation systems. This guideline also can serve as a reference for health care practitioners, health care facility managers, health care regulators, third-party payers, managed care organizations, consumers, and families. This document may be used in any of the following ways:

- To assist workers' compensation insurers, third-party administrators, self-insured corporations, and case management firms in understanding the services occupational therapists and occupational therapy assistants[1] can provide to clients on workers' compensation and the efficacy of these services in promoting return to work
- To assist occupational therapy practitioners in communicating about their services to external audiences, such as workers' compensation case managers and claims reviewers
- To assist physicians, other health care practitioners, employers, unions, and health care facility managers in determining whether referral for occupational therapy services would be appropriate
- To assist legislators, third-party payers, and administrators in understanding the professional education, training, and skills of occupational therapists and occupational therapy assistants relating to programs to improve work performance

---

[1] *Occupational therapists* are responsible for all aspects of occupational therapy service delivery and are accountable for the safety and effectiveness of the occupational therapy service delivery process. *Occupational therapy assistants* deliver occupational therapy services under the supervision of and in partnership with an occupational therapist (AOTA, 2009). When the term *occupational therapy practitioner* is used in this document, it refers to both occupational therapists and occupational therapy assistants (AOTA, 2006).

- To assist program developers, administrators, legislators, and third-party payers in understanding the scope of occupational therapy services
- To assist program evaluators and policy analysts in this practice area in determining outcome measures for analyzing the effectiveness of occupational therapy intervention
- To assist occupational therapy educators in designing appropriate curricula that incorporate the role of occupational therapy related to evaluation and intervention for clients with work-related injuries and populations of workers.

The introduction to this guideline continues with an overview of workers' compensation, the incidence of work-related injuries and illness, the importance of work in U.S. society, and a discussion of the domain and process of occupational therapy. The introduction is followed by a description of the occupational therapy process for assessment of and intervention with individuals having illnesses and/or injuries covered by workers' compensation. Next, a summary of the results of systematic reviews of evidence from the scientific literature presents best practices in occupational therapy intervention for individuals with clinical conditions and injuries typically involved in workers' compensation claims. Finally, appendixes contain the evidence-based literature review methodology, evidence tables, utilization guidelines, *CPT* coding, and additional information about occupational therapists and occupational therapy assistants.

Workers' Compensation

Workers' compensation is a system of benefits paid to workers who experience job-related injuries or illnesses. Benefits include medical expenses, rehabilitation, income replacement, permanent disability payments, and death benefits. Employers are required by law in all 50 states to provide workers' compensation benefits to their employees. Employers are responsible for payment regardless of fault; in return, the worker cannot sue the employer for the workplace conditions that contributed to the injury or illness.

Workers' compensation laws and provisions vary by state. These differences include method of administration, exemptions to certain categories of employees, medical benefits, physician selection, vocational rehabilitation, waiting periods, payment schedules, wage replacement benefits, and permanent disability benefits. Most states allow employers to buy workers' compensation policies directly from the state or a private insurer or to self-insure. A comparison of benefits by state is available at the Department of Labor's Web site at http://www. business.gov/business-law/employment/workers-compensation/state-workers-compensation.html.

Incidence of Work-Related Injuries and Illnesses

Work-related injuries and illnesses frequently result in functional loss, disability, and lost work time. In 2007 there were 4 million occupational injuries and illnesses in the United States, and 2 million of these led to lost work days, job transfer, or restrictions (U.S. Bureau of Labor Statistics, 2008). Over 40% of the injuries were sprains or strains, with most stemming from overexertion or falls on the same level. Musculoskeletal disorders accounted for more than 400,000 of the occupational illnesses requiring days away from work.

Occupational therapy practitioners are well prepared to assist this large population of individuals with work-related injuries and illnesses. Occupational therapy's primary role is to help individuals perform occupations and activities that are important to them. For individuals with work-related health problems, this may mean improving the strength of an injured limb to facilitate return to work, learning methods to manage symptoms on the job, performing job tasks in a safe manner, or problem solving at work to prevent future injuries or illnesses. Occupational therapists partner with employers to facilitate early return to work at a level of performance that is safe for the injured worker. Occupational therapy's focus on prevention of disability is a natural fit with the workers' compensation system.

Importance of Work

People have worked in one way or another since the beginnings of the human race. Work is integral to participation in society and provides many benefits to the worker. In addition to economic rewards, work provides meaning and fulfillment. Individuals develop self-confidence, skills, and competency through work. Engagement in work can promote quality of life and well-being. Work imposes structure on daily life and involves energy expenditure (Ruiz-Quintanilla & England, 1996).

Individuals who are eligible for workers' compensation continue to receive economic support through wage replacement; however, they lose the other health-promoting benefits that work provides. It is important to return injured workers to their jobs as soon as possible to prevent the negative consequences of prolonged time off from work. Research has demonstrated that depression (Keogh, Nuwayhid, Gordon, & Gucer, 2000), psychological distress (Feuerstein, Berkowitz, & Huang, 1999; Turner et al., 2007), weight gain (Cawley, 2000), and deconditioning (Musich, Napier, & Edington, 2001) are associated with loss of the worker role. Occupational therapy can help facilitate return to work and prevent the negative consequences of prolonged unemployment.

Domain and Process of Occupational Therapy

Occupational therapists' expertise lies in their knowledge of occupation and of how engaging in occupations can be used to improve human performance and ameliorate the effects of disease and disability (AOTA, 2008b). In 2002, the AOTA Representative Assembly adopted the *Occupational Therapy Practice Framework: Domain and Process* (AOTA, 2002). Informed by the previous *Uniform Terminology for Occupational Therapy* (AOTA, 1979, 1989, 1994) and the World Health Organization's (2001) *International Classification of Functioning, Disability, and Health*, the *Framework* outlines the profession's domain and the process of service delivery within this domain. The second edition of the *Occupational Therapy Practice Framework: Domain and Process* was published in 2008 (AOTA, 2008b).

Domain

A profession's domain articulates its members' sphere of knowledge, societal contribution, and intellectual or scientific activity. The occupational therapy profession's domain centers on helping others participate in daily life activities. The broad term that the profession uses to describe daily life activities is *occupation*. As outlined in the *Framework*, occupational therapists and occupational therapy assistants work collaboratively with clients to promote engagement in occupation to support participation in context or contexts, regardless of the practice setting or population (see Figure 1). This overarching mission circumscribes the profession's domain and emphasizes the important ways in which environmental and life circumstances influence how people carry out their occupations. Key aspects of the domain of occupational therapy are defined in Figure 2.

Process

Many professions use the process of evaluating, intervening, and targeting outcomes that is outlined in the *Framework*. Occupational therapy's application of this process is made unique, however, by its focus on occupation (see Figure 3). The process of occupational therapy service delivery begins with the *occupational profile;* an assessment of the client's occupational needs, problems, and concerns; and the *analysis of occupational performance*, which includes the performance skills, performance patterns, contexts, activity demands, and client factors that contribute to or impede the client's satisfaction with his or her ability to engage in valued daily life activities. Occupational therapists then plan and implement intervention using a variety of approaches and methods in which occupation is both the means and ends (Trombly, 1995). Occupational therapists continually assess the effectiveness of the intervention and the client's progress toward targeted

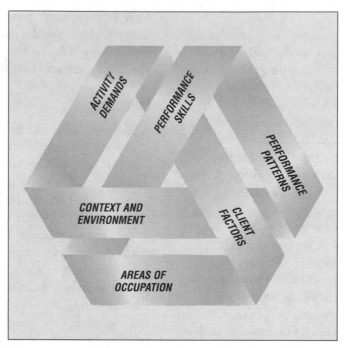

Figure 1. Occupational therapy's domain.

Source. From American Occupational Therapy Association. (2008). Occupational therapy practice framework: Domain and process (2nd ed., p. 627). *American Journal of Occupational Therapy, 62,* 625–683.

AREAS OF OCCUPATION	CLIENT FACTORS	PERFORMANCE SKILLS	PERFORMANCE PATTERNS	CONTEXT AND ENVIRONMENT	ACTIVITY DEMANDS
Activities of Daily Living (ADL)*	Values, Beliefs, and Spirituality	Sensory Perceptual Skills	Habits	Cultural	Objects Used and Their Properties
Instrumental Activities of Daily Living (IADL)	Body Functions	Motor and Praxis Skills	Routines	Personal	Space Demands
Rest and Sleep	Body Structures	Emotional Regulation Skills	Roles	Physical	Social Demands
Education		Cognitive Skills	Rituals	Social	Sequencing and Timing
Work		Communication and Social Skills		Temporal	Required Actions
Play				Virtual	Required Body Functions
Leisure					Required Body Structures
Social Participation?					
*Also referred to as *basic activities of daily living (BADL)* or *personal activities of daily living (PADL).*					

Figure 2. Aspects of occupational therapy's domain.

Source. From American Occupational Therapy Association. (2008). Occupational therapy practice framework: Domain and process (2nd ed., p. 628). *American Journal of Occupational Therapy, 62,* 625–683.

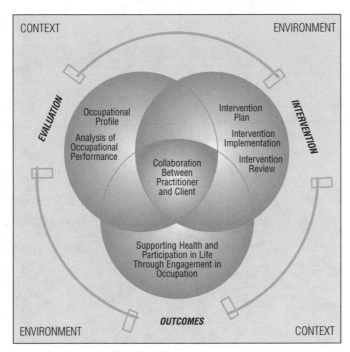

Figure 3. Occupational therapy's process.

Source. From American Occupational Therapy Association. (2008). Occupational therapy practice framework: Domain and process (2nd ed., p. 627). *American Journal of Occupational Therapy, 62,* 625–683.

outcomes. The *intervention review* informs decisions to continue or discontinue intervention and to make referrals to other agencies or professionals. Occupational therapists select outcome measures that are valid, reliable, and appropriately sensitive to the client's occupational performance, satisfaction, adaptation, role competence, health and wellness, prevention, and quality of life.

■ ■ ■

Occupational Therapy Process for Assessment and Treatment of Individuals With Work-Related Injuries and Illnesses

Occupational therapists and occupational therapy assistants in a diverse array of settings work with individuals who have sustained work-related injuries and illnesses. The most common setting is an outpatient setting at a hospital or clinic in the community. Frequently, occupational therapy practitioners encounter such clients in occupational medicine and rehabilitation clinics that provide functional capacity evaluations (FCEs), work hardening, work conditioning, and ergonomic services. However, occupational therapy treatment may begin during the inpatient hospital stay, as early as in the intensive care unit. In addition, in-home occupational therapy services may be provided to clients who are not able to travel to the outpatient setting. Still other services are provided at the work site; clients transitioning back to work benefit from on-the-job occupational therapy services to identify the safest work methods, perform activity and environmental modifications, and monitor symptom management.

The referral and evaluation processes vary depending on the setting; however, occupational therapy practice in all settings focuses on engagement in everyday life activities that are meaningful to the client. For clients with work-related injuries or illnesses, work performance is the priority. The occupational therapist considers both factors intrinsic to the client (perfor-

mance skills, body functions, body structures) and extrinsic factors (work environment, requirements of the job) important for work performance. The focus of intervention is on the functional abilities of the worker to perform the job demands, implement adaptations, and develop habits and routines that support successful work performance.

The occupational therapy process is similar across settings. This process begins with referral and evaluation, moves on to intervention, and ends with post-intervention planning and follow-up.

Initiation of Occupational Therapy Services

Interruption of a client's occupational performance can have many detrimental effects. Many clients begin to see themselves as "patients" whose role is to rest, take medication, and do stretching exercises. Therefore, it is important to help a client with a work-related injury or illness stay connected to his or her many roles, including the worker role. As soon as medically appropriate, the client should begin occupational therapy. The focus of assessment and treatment initially may be performance of daily self-care skills, but it will soon progress to performance of home, community, and work activities.

Work assessment can begin as soon as medically feasible. If the client has been in the patient role for an extended period, it may be difficult for him or her to envision resuming the worker role. The client must make this paradigm shift to succeed in work rehabilitation. Early work assessment will identify the client's work capacities to facilitate resumption of partial or restricted work duties at a level that is safe for the client. If a client begins work-focused occupational therapy early, the worker role will be maintained, and return to work will be easier. In some cases, the client may be able to return to work after the initial work assessment with only minor job accommodations. In other cases, the client must participate in an occupational therapy treatment program to achieve the tolerance levels needed to safely return to work.

Clients with limitations in their work performance are typically referred to the occupational therapist for evaluation and intervention. At times the referral may be for specific services, such as a functional capacity evaluation, work hardening, or work conditioning. The referral source should provide information including reason for referral, medical diagnosis, current treatment, medical clearance and restrictions, and current medications. In most states, the employer, insurance company, or client initiates the referral to occupational therapy. However, the occupational therapy practice act in many states requires a referral for occupational therapy services from a licensed physician or other health care professional. Several states require a physician's referral for treatment but not for occupational therapy evaluation or for prevention or ergonomic consultation.

In states where a physician referral is not required, many occupational therapy settings require a physician's referral to meet third-party payer requirements. Some settings require insurance preauthorization. Workers' compensation statutes and insurance requirements may also require a referral for services. If occupational therapy is being provided at the work site, the referral requirements dictated by the state occupational therapy practice act must be followed. The following are some common sources of referral for occupational therapy services:

- Physicians of varying specialties, including but not limited to general practitioners, occupational medicine practitioners, physiatrists, orthopedists, neurologists, osteopaths, family medicine practitioners, internists, sports medicine practitioners, and psychiatrists
- Case managers
- Employers
- Employee health nurses
- Employer safety representatives
- Human resource professionals
- Workers' compensation insurance carriers
- Third-party payers
- Other rehabilitation providers
- Psychologists
- Social workers
- Vocational evaluators and counselors
- Attorneys
- Chiropractic physicians.

Clients may self-refer in some states where a physician referral is not required.

Evaluation

The occupational therapist performs the evaluation in collaboration with the client on the basis of targeted information specific to the desired outcomes. The two elements of the occupational therapy evaluation are (a) the occupational profile and (b) the analysis of occupational performance (AOTA, 2008b). The occupational therapy evaluation process for a client with a work-related injury or illness is multidimensional. To establish a collaborative therapeutic relationship with the client early in the evaluation process, the occupational therapist first identifies the client's priorities to help guide the initial assessment. The desired outcome of treatment—engagement in work performance—serves as the focus of and drives the evaluation process.

Occupational therapists use a variety of assessment methods to perform the work performance evaluation, including client interview, observation, rating scales, questionnaires, diagrams, manual testing, performance testing, and work simulations. The occupational therapist may administer both standardized and non-standardized assessments. Some assessments are compared to normative data, and others are compared to criterion-referenced data, namely the requirements of the job and the work setting. To understand the work environment and job demands, the occupational therapist uses a variety of assessment methods, including client interview, employer interview, job site analysis, and job description review and refers to national job data such as that provided by the Occupational Information Network (http://online.onetcenter.org/).

The occupational therapy evaluation of a client with a work-related injury or illness is both client centered and job specific. The assessment of factors both intrinsic and extrinsic to the client provides the occupational therapist with a thorough understanding of the client's ability to function on the job (the client in his or her work context). The occupational therapist must ensure that any assessment instrument used is safe, reliable, and valid, a necessity in the highly litigious workers' compensation environment. The goal of the evaluation is to develop a fair and accurate understanding of the client's present work performance, potential to return to work, and interventions indicated to prepare for resumption of work duties.

Occupational Profile

The occupational therapist develops an occupational profile to gain an understanding of the client's perspective and background. Through both formal interviews and informal conversations, the occupational therapist learns what is currently important and meaningful to the client and identifies past experiences and interests that may contribute to the client's current issues and problems. The purpose of developing the occupational profile is to determine who the client or clients are, identify their needs or concerns, and ascertain how these concerns affect engagement in occupational performance. Developing the occupational profile involves the following steps:

- *Identify the client or clients.* The individual with the work-related injury is the ultimate client in all cases; however, the physician, insurance company, and employer are also clients of occupational therapy services. The goals of these clients may vary, but the occupational therapist considers all perspectives.
- *Determine why the client is seeking services.* Through interviews or checklists, the occupational therapist assists the client in identifying his or her current concerns relative to the areas of occupation and performance.
- *Identify the areas of occupation that are successful and the areas in which the client is experiencing problems.* On the basis of the client's current concerns, the occupational therapist identifies possible barriers and supports related to occupational performance.
- *Discuss significant aspects of the client's occupational history.* The client's life experiences, including medical interventions, employment history, vocational preferences, community roles, interests, and previous patterns of engagement in occupations, shape how the person deals with everyday routines and occupations.
- *Determine the client's priorities and desired outcomes.* Before intervention occurs, the therapist and client discuss and prioritize outcomes so that the therapist's evaluation and intervention will match the client's desired goals (outcomes). The therapist may need to refer the client to other professionals to achieve these outcomes.

Analysis of Occupational Performance

The occupational therapist uses information from the occupational profile to focus on the specific areas of occupation and the context to be addressed. The following steps are generally included in analyzing occupational performance:

- *Observe the client* as he or she performs the occupations in the natural or least restrictive environment (when possible), and note the effectiveness of the client's performance skills (e.g., motor and praxis, sensory–perceptual, emotional regulation, cognitive, communication and social) and performance patterns (e.g., habits, routines, roles).

- *Select specific assessments and assessment methods* that will identify and measure the factors related to the specific aspects of the domain influencing the client's performance.
- *Interpret the assessment data* to identify what supports or hinders performance.
- *Develop or refine a hypothesis* regarding the client's performance.
- If intervention is indicated, *develop goals in collaboration with the client* that address the client's desired outcomes. The desired outcome of work performance as previously performed may or may not be possible.
- *Identify potential intervention approaches*, guided by best practice and the evidence, and discuss them with the client.
- *Document the evaluation process*, and communicate the results to the appropriate team members and community agencies. Interested parties may include the physician, the employer, workers' compensation insurance personnel, and the case manager.

Areas of Occupation

The main occupation of concern for clients with work-related injuries is work performance. However, the client's performance in other areas of occupation, such as driving, home maintenance, and leisure tasks, can affect the client's overall well-being and capacity to perform work tasks. Therefore, the occupational therapist may discuss or observe performance of these tasks during the evaluation process.

The occupational therapist gathers predictive evaluation data regarding the client's ability to return to work primarily through work performance testing. The therapist usually observes simulated or actual performance of work activities (tasks) after he or she has evaluated the client's body structures, body functions, and performance skills and understands the requirements of the job. The therapist must understand the client's current impairments to ensure that

the client's safety is maintained throughout the assessment. These impaired functions may not necessarily be directly related to the current work-related injury, but they may be critical for safe work performance. For example, if a client with a neck injury also has sensory loss in the lower extremities because of diabetes, he may not have adequate neck flexion to use his previous technique of observing where he positions his foot on the rung of a ladder to compensate for decreased sensation; hence, it may not be safe for the client to climb a ladder.

The occupational therapist closely monitors the client's tolerance for an activity and makes incremental increases in the work demands until the client reaches his or her maximum safe level of performance. The therapist observes the client's work habits and ability to compensate for impairments and to manage his or her pain or other symptoms. The impact of the client's impairments in body functions and performance skills on his or her ability to perform job tasks will become apparent during work performance testing, as will the client's habits and routines.

Performance Skills

The occupational therapist evaluates overt and subtle factors that may affect work performance. *Performance skills* are the abilities clients demonstrate in the actions they perform: "Occupational therapy practitioners observe and analyze performance skills in order to understand the transactions among underlying factors that support or hinder engagement in occupations and occupational performance" (AOTA, 2008b, p. 639). The five types of performance skills are motor and praxis, sensory–perceptual, emotional regulation, cognitive, and communication and social skills.

Performance skills are closely linked and are used in combination with one another to allow the client to perform an occupation. The client's level of competency and skill performance must match the skill level required of the job. The occupational therapist first understands the job requirements and then designs the evaluation to assess essential performance skills. For example, if an individual is an electrician recuperating from a foot injury and resultant pain disorder, testing focuses heavily on motor and praxis skills, such as walking, climbing, balancing, and squatting. If this client has problems focusing and attending to tasks because of pain or the side effects of medication, the therapist tests the client's cognitive skills. If this client experiences problems with frustration tolerance that spill over into interactions with others, emotional regulation may need to be assessed. Table 1 summarizes the performance skill areas and provides work-related examples.

Client Factors

Client factors are specific abilities, characteristics, or beliefs that reside within the client and may affect performance in areas of occupation (AOTA, 2008b). The client factors include body functions; body structures; and the client's values, beliefs, and spirituality. These underlying client factors are affected by the presence or absence of illness, disease, deprivation, and disability. The client factors support the performance skills.

Body functions refer to the "physiological function of body systems (including psychological functions)" (World Health Organization [WHO], 2001, p. 10). *Body structures* are the "anatomical parts of the body such as organs, limbs, and their components" (WHO, 2001, p. 10). Body structures and body functions are interrelated (e.g., the heart and blood vessels are body

Table 1. Performance Skills and Selected Work-Related Examples

Performance Skills	Examples
Motor and praxis skills	Bending and reaching for a tool in a storage closet Pacing tempo of movements to clean the workroom Coordinating body movements to complete a job task Maintaining balance while walking on an uneven outdoor surface or working on a ladder Anticipating or adjusting posture and body position in response to environmental circumstances, such as varying height levels Manipulating equipment parts
Cognitive skills	Selecting the tools and supplies needed to keep the work area clean Sequencing tasks needed to plan for a conference presentation Organizing activities within the time required to meet a deadline Prioritizing steps and identifying solutions to pick up multiple truckloads from a vendor Multitasking—doing more than one task at a time at work
Communication and social skills	Looking where someone else is pointing or gazing Gesturing to emphasize intentions Maintaining acceptable physical space during conversation Initiating and answering questions with relevant information when preparing for a presentation at work Taking turns during an interchange with another person verbally and physically Acknowledging a coworker's perspective during an interchange
Sensory–perceptual skills	Knowing where the foot is in space in relationship to the foot pedal and sensing the amount of pressure needed to engage pedal to desired level Identifying noxious fumes in a factory setting Hearing and locating the voice of a coworker in a crowd Visually determining the correct size of a storage container for leftover books Locating keys by touch from many objects in a work tote bag (i.e., stereognosis) Timing the appropriate moment to cross the street when going from one facility to another by determining one's own position and speed relative to the speed of traffic
Emotional-regulation skills	Responding to the feelings of coworkers by acknowledgment or show of support Persisting in a task despite frustrations Controlling anger toward customers and coworkers and avoiding aggressive acts Displaying emotions that are appropriate for the situation Using relaxation strategies to cope with stressful events

structures that support cardiovascular functions such as blood pressure). Activity demands vary greatly among jobs, but most jobs require emotional, cognitive, sensory, and motor functioning. Therefore, the occupational therapist may evaluate the body structures—for example, the integrity of the structures in a joint or the response of a nerve to tapping or stretching. The related body functions may include the capacity of the knee to maintain stability when carrying a heavy load or the ability to manipulate objects despite tingling in the fingers. The body functions may need thorough evaluation or a simple screen, depending on the client and the potential effect of these functions on the client's ability to work. Body functions within the occupational therapy practitioner's domain of practice and work-related examples are outlined in Table 2.

Table 2. Body Functions and Selected Work-Related Examples

Body Functions	Specific Functions	Examples
Mental functions	Temperament and personality functions	Conscientiousness in communication with coworker, maintaining emotional stability when frustrated, openness to experience
	Energy and drive function	Motivation to continue despite problems, impulse control with angry customer, interests and values relative to work
	Attention functions	Sustained attention to complete quality review, dividing attention between talking on the phone and doing a paperwork task
	Memory functions	Retrospective memory of how work issues were handled, prospective memory to perform a work task in the future, working memory to recall threshold while performing quality control
	Perceptual functions	Visuospatial perceptions to place part into automobile, interpretation of sensory stimuli to feel heartbeat of artery (e.g., tactile, visual, auditory), temporal relationships allowing for timely return from work breaks, multisensory processing of multimodal input in a factory environment
	Thought functions	Recognition of customers, categorization of expenses into correct category, logical and coherent thought when making decision, appropriate thought content for the workplace setting
	Higher level cognitive functions	Judgment to avoid inappropriate relationships with coworkers, making decisions about how to handle a customer, managing time to complete task per schedule, problem solving to meet staffing needs, metacognition, cognitive flexibility, insight, maintaining attention during staff meeting, awareness of the effect of tardiness
	Mental functions of language	Ability to understand language and express oneself during interactions with customer
	Calculation functions	Ability to balance the cash register drawer
	Functions to sequence complex movement	Planning movements to climb a ladder
	Psychomotor functions	Appropriate range and regulation of motor response to psychological events
	Emotional functions	Displaying appropriate emotions for the situation, ability to regulate emotions regarding personal relationships while at the workplace, control of anger while receiving feedback from supervisor
	Experience of self and time functions	Body image, accurate self-concept of abilities, self-esteem to do tasks correctly

Table 2. Body Functions and Selected Work-Related Examples *(cont.)*

Body Functions	Specific Functions	Examples
Sensory functions and pain	Touch functions	Ability to sense pressure needed to push keyboard, ability to discriminate where to insert bolt in engine compartment
	Position in space functions	Proprioception, kinesthesia
	Vision functions	Visual acuity allowing proper viewing of gauges in cockpit, visual field functions allowing for view of the entire playground of children
	Hearing functions	Response to sound such as an alarm or the rattle in an automobile
	Vestibular function	Balancing while walking on roof of house
	Other sensory functions	Tasting the sauce for salt, smelling alcohol on a driver's breath, sensing temperature of a baby
	Sensations of pain	Ability to discriminate types of pain and pain intensity to avoid injury at work
Neuromusculoskeletal and movement-related functions	Functions of joints and bones	Mobility of joints and bones allowing for reaching the overhead shelf, stability of joints, postural alignment of the soldier standing at attention
	Muscle functions	Power burst to remove a motorcycle from the injured driver, strength to lift window into place, muscle endurance to load a truck with wood boards
	Movement functions	Reflexes to remove finger from hot stove, eye–hand/foot coordination to operate overhead crane, bilateral integration needed to control a squirming newborn baby, controlling involuntary movements to avoid accidentally turning steering wheel, gait pattern of a model on the runway
Cardiovascular functions		Blood pressure, heart rate, and rhythm within normal range to allow for endurance to work
Respiratory functions		Respiration rate, rhythm, and oxygenation within normal range to allow for endurance to work
Other supportive functions	Exercise tolerance functions	Aerobic capacity allowing a bicycle delivery person to complete the route, stamina of a hockey player, physical endurance to walk to parking lot
	Skin functions	Protective functions of the skin, wound healing, and nail health for safe handling of food items
	Hematological, immunological, genitourinary, digestive, metabolic, voice/speech functions	Depending on setting, the occupational therapy practitioner may have expertise in these functions.

Note. Some data adapted from the *Occupational Therapy Practice Framework* (AOTA, 2008b) and the *International Classification of Functioning, Disability, and Health* (WHO, 2001).

Performance Patterns

Performance patterns "refer to habits, routines, roles, and rituals used in the process of engaging in occupations or activities" (AOTA, 2008b, p. 641). Performance patterns help occupational therapy practitioners understand the frequency and manner in which performance skills and occupations are integrated into the client's life. Adaptive habits and routines may help a client compensate for impairments in body functions and performance skills. For example, a client who is habitually late for appointments may not be competitive in the workforce; however, use of an electronic planner with an alarm may be an effective compensatory method.

During the evaluation process, the occupational therapist begins to identify habits and routines that are useful and detrimental to the client in the workforce.

The therapist seeks to understand the client's performance patterns and to formulate a more accurate assessment of the impact of these performance patterns on work performance by observing the sequences and patterns of the client's routines and habits. When a client is involved in an intervention program, the therapist will have more opportunities to observe the client's routines and habits and assess their effect on work performance.

Context and Environment

Context "refers to a variety of interrelated conditions that are within and surrounding the client" (AOTA, 2008b, p. 642) that exert a strong influence on performance; "the term *environment* refers to the external physical and social environments that surround the client and in which the client's daily life occupations occur" (AOTA, 2008b, p. 642). Occupational therapists acknowledge the influence of cultural, personal, temporal, and virtual contextual factors and physical and social environmental factors on occupations and activities. The context and environment have a strong effect on the client's performance as he or she prepares to return to work. A strong cultural push to return to work, coworkers and supervisors willing to assist with the return-to-work process, and a physical environment that supports the client's work adaptations will help propel the client back to work. Alternatively, maladaptive contexts and environments, such as an attorney's advice to stay off work as long as possible and economic rewards from work disability policies and benefits, may prevent the client from returning to work. The occupational therapist considers the client's contexts and environments during the assessment and throughout intervention with clients with work-related injuries and illnesses.

Cultural Factors

The evaluation process should include awareness of the client's cultural beliefs and behaviors regarding work. The occupational therapist should identify beliefs or client information that is critical to a successful return to work. A strong work ethic may keep a client at the workplace even when the work tasks aggravate a medical condition for which the healing process requires rest. The culture of the workplace also influences whether an intervention plan is acceptable to both the client and employer; a workplace that easily accommodates employees with work restrictions and treats them as valuable members of the work team will provide the support an injured worker needs to both recover from the injury and maintain the worker role.

Personal Factors

Some client personal attributes, such as gender, socioeconomic status, age, and level of education, should be factored into the evaluation process. For example, an older worker who is recovering from a work-related injury may demonstrate age-related strength deficits in addition to the impairments resulting from the injury. A worker with many financial commitments may feel pressured to return to work earlier than recommended to avoid losing his or her automobile or home. The occupational therapist must ensure that the assessment is not discriminatory due to use of age- or gender-driven norms or differences in testing protocols on the basis of personal attributes.

Temporal Factors

The occupational therapist must consider the temporal context when working with a client recovering from a work-related injury or illness. On the client level, *temporal context* may refer to the point in the person's life span. For example, a younger worker may be able to learn a new skill or change employers if unable to meet the demands of the current job, whereas an older worker may have fewer options regarding job change.

Temporal context also may refer to the point in the progression of or recovery from an injury or disease, such as the preventive, acute, or rehabilitative phase or the long-term process of dealing with a chronic illness. The needs of a client taking measures to improve the ergonomic setup of the workstation to prevent carpal tunnel syndrome differ from those of a client experiencing long-term impairments from chronic carpal tunnel syndrome.

On a smaller scale, *temporal context* refers to the amount of time the client is capable of participating in the evaluation. The occupational therapist can make a more accurate appraisal of a client's ability to work if the assessment schedule simulates the normal work schedule. A client may be able to perform a simulated work task for a 2-hour interval without any difficulty but may not be able to tolerate this task for an entire 8-hour work shift or back-to-back days, as is required at work.

Virtual Factors

Interface with the virtual environment is required at some workplaces; therefore, occupational therapists in rehabilitation settings may assess related skills. Many workers are required to use virtual communication through airways or computers to substitute for physical contact (AOTA, 2008b). They may navigate the Internet and communicate via e-mail, videoconferencing, or radio transmissions. The therapist may use similar technologies to assess the client's ability to use the workplace virtual environment. In addition, occupational therapists may use work simulation equipment, driving simulators, and other virtual technology during rehabilitation to assess the client's performance skills and simulate job demands.

Physical Factors

The physical environment must be considered during the evaluation and treatment process. The physical environment at the workplace must be conducive to the client's recovery. For example, a client with an open burn needs to be in a clean environment for healing to occur, or a client who is now required to use a wheelchair or walker needs to be in an accessible workplace. During the clinic-based assessment, the therapist may be able to simulate some characteristics of the physical work environment to make a more accurate assessment of the client's capacity to work, such as matching the height of a shelf a client must lift to or simulating the noise level to assess ability to attend amid distractions. To ensure a successful return to work, the physical environment at the workplace may need to be modi-fied to support the client's performance within his or her capacities. The occupational therapist is well prepared to analyze the workplace and make appropriate environmental modifications to support work performance.

Social Factors

Many social factors in the home, community, rehabilitation setting, and work site affect recovery. During rehabilitation, the client's relationships with the physician, rehabilitation team, case manager, insurance company, and employer are important, as are the client's social interactions in the family and community. For example, a client's spouse can encourage regular therapy participation and performance of a home activity program or, alternatively, can discourage return to work by talking negatively about the employer. A supportive employer who is willing to problem-solve with the client and the therapist to ensure a smooth transition to the workplace provides a positive social context for the client. The occupational therapist in collaboration with the rehabilitation case manager can facilitate communication among the individuals in the client's social environment.

Activity Demands

Activity demands refer to the specific features of a task that influence the type and amount of effort required to perform the activity (AOTA, 2008b). The occupational therapist must understand the demands of the various activities that make up the client's job to make an accurate assessment of the client's ability to work. These factors may include the work tasks that the client performs; work procedures and processes; productivity expectations; the design of the work space; the equipment, materials, and tools used on the job; time demands; and the skills and functions required to perform job tasks. The occupational therapist uses information about the job to guide aspects of the evaluation process such as simulating the work environment, work pace, and work tasks and selecting the required performance skills and body functions to be evaluated.

The therapist uses several methods to identify the job demands (essential job functions), including interviews with the client, discussion with the employer, review of the employer's written job description, and analysis of the job at the work site (job analysis). The therapist must collaborate with the employer to get the most detailed job analysis possible. The therapist may refer to the Department of Labor's Occupational Information Network (http://online.onetcenter.org) to find generic job descriptions. If the client will not return to his or her previous job, the therapist can use these generic resources to explore potential jobs. The therapist may borrow equipment and tools used on the job from the employer to help simulate the job requirements.

Considerations in Using Assessments

The occupational therapist designs an assessment battery that is tailored to meet the individual needs of the client. Each assessment in the battery should be safe, reliable, valid, and practical according to the National Institute for Occupational Safety and Health (NIOSH, 1981).

Legal and Professional Guidelines and Standards

The occupational therapist follows all national and state guidelines that govern assessment in occupational therapy. When decisions affecting employment are being made, the therapist must adhere to the federal guidelines for employee testing described in the *Uniform Guidelines for Employee Selection* (U.S. Department of Labor, 1978). These guidelines require that a test not discriminate on the basis of gender, race, or age. When testing individuals with disabilities, the therapist must comply with the Americans With Disabilities Act (ADA; 1990). The therapist must make reasonable accommodations during the assessment, including allowing use of mobility devices, assistive technology, and modified testing methods. Although these accommodations may decrease the reliability of the test, they will ensure the safety of the client and improve the usefulness of the results. The U.S. Department of Labor Web site

describes many employment laws (http://www.dol.gov/compliance/laws/main.htm).

Occupational therapists should follow the *Occupational Therapy Practice Framework* when performing assessments, including work assessments (AOTA, 2008b). In addition, occupational therapists may adhere to guidelines from other professional organizations when performing a work evaluation, such as the guidelines developed jointly by the American Educational Research Association, the American Psychological Association, and the National Council on Measurement in Education (1999) and those of the American Congress of Sports Medicine (Whaley, Brubaker, & Otto, 2006).

The Functional Assessment Network (2003), affiliated with McMaster University in Hamilton, Ontario, Canada, has developed guidelines for the assessment of individuals with work-related injuries. This network's guidelines address assessments that measure a client's ability to perform work. The guidelines apply to a full spectrum of stakeholder groups in Canada, including workers and worker representatives, state insurance boards, employers, other types of insurance payers, clinicians who perform work evaluations, health care providers, labor, research and academia, and government. The Functional Assessment Network recommends an individualized systematic testing protocol over a 2-day period that includes self-report, observation, standardized instruments, and functional or work simulation tasks. The network also recommends that assessment be driven by clinical reasoning and be sufficiently challenging to match the actual demands of the job and to capture optimal performance that may not be sustainable in full-time work (http://www.fhs.mcmaster.ca/rehab/FA%20Guidelines.pdf).

Guidelines and Standards for Safety, Reliability, and Validity

In order to meet NIOSH criteria for the development and selection of work-related assessments, the assessment must demonstrate safety, reliability, validity, practicality, and utility (Innes & Straker, 2003). The following hierarchical framework for testing derived from these guidelines and standards is very useful when performing work assessment (Matheson, 2003):

1. *Safety*—The client's safety must be the first priority of the therapist throughout the assessment.
2. *Reliability*—The results should be consistent across therapists and clients and from one time to the next.
3. *Validity*—The results should reflect the client's true ability.
4. *Practicality*—The costs, interpretation, and reporting should be reasonable and useful.

As with all hierarchies, criteria toward the top of the list are more important than those lower on the list. Therefore, if the test instrument has high reliability but the safety of the client cannot be maintained throughout the assessment, the results are not meaningful.

Safety During the Work Assessment

The occupational therapist's first priority during the work assessment is to ensure the safety of the client. The assessment must not subject the client to physical, sensory, or emotional harm. Because these clients are recuperating from injuries or illnesses, they may have impaired body structures and functions, and therefore they may experience pain or fatigue or be susceptible to injury or exacerbation of symptoms. For example, a client who underwent a two-level spinal fusion experiences structural changes that decrease spine range of motion and trunk flexibility. The therapist must bear in mind that when the client is performing bending and lifting tasks, he or she may experience pain in muscles that are deconditioned or may move excessively at other levels of the spine to make up for the limited mobility at the level of the fusion.

The occupational therapist reviews medical records, interviews the client, and screens the body structures and functions to ensure safety before evaluating the client's ability to perform work tasks. This screen varies depending on the client's status and history but may include assessment of sensory functions, mental functions, balance and stability, and cardiovascular functions. Further testing may be indicated if problems are identified. The therapist progresses with testing only if the assessment can follow the precautions identified during screening and any restrictions imposed by the referring physician. The therapist monitors the client's condition closely during testing, including heart rate, symptoms (e.g., pain, numbness, other sensations the client self-reports), movement patterns, body mechanics, and fatigue. Because obesity can stress the cardiopulmonary and musculoskeletal systems, the therapist diligently monitors clients who are obese or in poor physical condition.

Reliability of the Work Assessment

Once the safety of the assessment has been addressed, reliability is the next important consideration. *Reliability* is the extent to which the assessment is consistent and free of error. Types of reliability include the following (Portney & Watkins, 2008):

- *Test–retest reliability*—Consistency of results if the assessment is administered repeatedly
- *Intrarater reliability*—Consistency of results achieved by the same rater over more than one occasion
- *Interrater reliability*—Consistency of results when two or more evaluators administer the assessment to the same participant
- *Internal consistency*—Consistency of the assessment in measuring the various aspects of the same characteristics.

Reliability depends not only on properties of the instrument but also on the occupational therapist's competency in administering it. Use of standardized testing methods will ensure that the assessment results are reliable and reproducible. Reliable results are especially important when performing a work assessment because the client must be able to dependably perform job tasks on a day-to-day basis. When using standardized instruments, the therapist follows the assessment protocol outlined in the administration manual. The therapist ensures that equipment and instruments used during the assessment are calibrated and maintained. The therapist also provides specific directions to the client and ensures that he or she understands what is expected before beginning the assessment to ensure that the client's performance is reliable during the assessment. The therapist monitors the client's response and uses clinical reasoning to ensure that the client's safety is maintained during testing.

Reliability of the Client: Role of Maximal Effort in Testing

An important aspect of reliability is the client's need to perform at his or her maximum safe capacity, known as *maximal effort,* during the work assessment. The occupational therapist explains this to the client before each test that requires maximal effort to ensure that the client understands that the reliability of his or her effort is being monitored. The concept of maximal effort may be novel to most clients recuperating from illness or injury. Many of these clients have been under activity restrictions or have been told to limit their performance to minimize pain while recovering from their illness or injury. Therefore, clients may be anxious about giving maximal effort because they fear reinjury.

The occupational therapist helps the client understand that the objective of performance testing is to identify his or her present tolerance level for various activities so the therapist can develop the best plan to compensate for or remediate performance deficits. Before initiating maximal effort testing, the therapist addresses the client's concerns to help alleviate anxiety and ensures that the client understands the requirements of the assessment. If the therapist notes inconsistencies in the client's performance or signs that the client did not provide maximal effort on a test in the battery, the therapist may explain his or her specific observations and explore possible reasons with the client. Most likely the reason for inconsistent effort is fear, anxiety, pain, fatigue, or decreased physical fitness. Rarely does a client purposefully mask his or her real abilities; malingering syndrome has been shown to be rare (Leavitt & Sweet, 1986). Again, the therapist always places safety as a top priority over the reliability of the test protocol or ability of the client to provide consistent maximal effort during the assessment.

Validity of the Work Assessment

Validity refers to the extent to which an assessment tests what it is intended to measure. According to Portney and Watkins (2008), because a valid measure is relatively free from error, a valid instrument also would be reliable. Types of measurement validity include the following:

- *Face validity* indicates that the test seems to measure what it should.
- *Content validity* establishes whether the test assesses the domains it claims to measure; this can be done by a consensus of experts who determine that the items included in the measure adequately sample the universe of content.
- *Concurrent validity* establishes validity when two measures are taken at the same time, and one is considered to be the gold standard for assessment in a given area.
- *Predictive validity* indicates how well a measure predicts future performance on a criterion variable.
- *Construct validity* reflects whether an instrument adequately measures a theoretical construct (Portney & Watkins, 2008).

A work assessment must be able to discriminate between a client who can safely perform his or her job and a client who is not able to perform the required job duties. A standardized assessment may have excellent reliability; however, validity may be limited because the equipment, methods, and pace of performance are usually dictated by the testing protocol. Therefore, the occupational therapist uses job-specific tasks, methods, and equipment to ensure that the assessment replicates the job as closely as possible. The therapist collaborates with the employer to get the tools and equipment needed to make the assessment as real to life as possible. For example, the therapist may request to use the actual pry bar fabricated in the employer's metal shop or the scanning gun a clerk uses. The therapist will not be able to simulate all of the unique demands of the work tasks and the work environment in a clinic setting; if possible, portions of the assessment can be performed at the work site. Again, the occupational therapist focuses on safety first, then reliability, and then validity while performing the work assessment.

Practicality

The costs of the assessment, time to schedule and complete the assessment, and reporting turn-around time should be reasonable. The results in the evaluation report should be easily interpreted and answer the referral question.

Standardized Evaluation Instruments and Batteries

Sample assessments that are potentially useful in work evaluations are listed in Table 3. Standardized assessments require a methodical process of administration and result in quantifiable information that compares to a norm group or a specific criterion, and research is usually available to demonstrate that the assessment actually is measuring what it claims to assess (validity). Therapists using standardized assessments must follow the procedure outlined in the administration manual and interpret the results as instructed, including ensuring that the client is similar to the norm group in age, diagnosis, and setting or that the reference criterion is accurate for the client's situation. Some standardized assessments require or recommend that the therapist attend training and/or obtain certification to use the instrument.

Nonstandardized assessments allow for flexibility during administration, can be designed to match the specific job requirements, and result in more qualitative information. Because there are thousands of different jobs in the U.S. economy, standardized performance assessments at the occupation-based level rarely exist, and the few that do exist are not accessible to most therapists because they were developed to screen new hires for a particular employer.

Most standardized assessments that measure work performance at the occupation-based level use client self-report or generic productivity estimations. There has been conflicting evidence regarding the correlation between self-report measures and actual abilities, but

self-report measures help the therapist understand the client's perceptions of his or her abilities before actual performance testing. When testing individuals with chronic low back pain, administration of performance-based and self-report assessments is recommended (Reneman, Dijkstra, Westmaas, & Göeken, 2002). Job-specific performance testing is usually performed using job simulations; however, the therapist may use a standardized method for administering these job simulations. All measurable aspects of the client's performance should be quantified so the therapist can compare the client's abilities to the essential job functions. The therapist should also gather qualitative data to describe the client's work methods and response to the work task.

The occupational therapist may use a standardized work assessment battery to measure the client's performance skill and body functions. Several batteries that measure work performance at this level exist; they are typically referred to as *functional capacity evaluations (FCEs)*. A panel of international experts recently identified two definitions for FCE. The first is "an evaluation designed to document and to describe a person's current safe work ability from a physical ability and motivational perspective with consideration given to any existing medical, impairment, and/or pain syndromes" (Soer, van der Schans, Groothoff, Geertzen, & Reneman, 2008, p. 394). The second is "an evaluation of capacity of activities that is used to make recommendations for participation in work while considering the person's body functions and structures, environmental factors, personal factors, and health status" (Soer et al., 2008, p. 394). The performance skills and body functions typically assessed in these batteries include mobility, strength (static and dynamic), material handling (lifting, carrying, pushing, and pulling), tolerance of positions and movements, and cardiovascular fitness (Legge & Burgess-Limerick, 2007).

The reliability and validity of several FCE batteries have been established. Innes (2006) reviewed the reliability and validity of FCEs and found that the Isernhagen/WorkWell System has the most peer-reviewed evidence for reliability and validity, including interrater

Table 3. Examples of Selected Assessments

Area of Evaluation	Assessment	Reference
Areas of occupation	Disabilities of the Arm, Shoulder, and Head	Hudak et al., 1996
	Functional Abilities Confidence Scale	Williams & Myers, 1998
	Hand Function Sort	Matheson, Kaskutas, & Mada, 2001
	Occupational Role Questionnaire	Kopec & Esdaile, 1998
	Oswestry Low Back Pain Disability Questionnaire	Fairbank, Couper, Davies, & O'Brien, 1980
	Patient-Related Wrist and Hand	MacDermid, Turgeon, Richards, Beadle, & Roth, 1998
	Roland Morris Disability Questionnaire	Roland & Morris, 1983
	Spinal Function Sort	Matheson, Matheson, & Grant, 1993
	Vermont Disability Questionnaire	Hazard, Haugh, Reid, Preble, & McDonald, 1996
	Work Ability Index	Karazman, Kloimuller, Geissler, & Karazman-Morawetz, 1999
	Work Instability Scale	Gilworth et al., 2003
	Work Limitations Questionnaire	Lerner et al., 2001
	Work Productivity and Impairment Questionnaire	Reilly, Zbrozek, & Dukes, 1993
	Work Role Functioning Questionnaire	Lerner, Malspeis, Rogers, & Amick, 1995
Activity demands	Occupational Information Network (O*NET)— The Department of Labor's online database describing jobs in the U.S. economy	http://online.onetcenter.org/
	Revised NIOSH Lifting Equation	NIOSH, 1994
	Strain Index	Moore & Garg, 1995
	OSHA Screening Tool: VDT Checklist	OSHA, 2000
	Rapid Upper Limb Assessment	McAtamney & Corlett, 1993
	Liberty Mutual Material Handling Guidelines	Liberty Mutual, 2004
	Rapid Entire Body Assessment	Hignett & McAtamney, 2000
	ACGIH TLV® for Hand Activity Level	ACGIH Worldwide, 2002
Context and environment	Job Content Questionnaire	Karasek et al., 1998
	Job Requirements and Physical Demands Survey	Marcotte, Barker, Joyce, Miller, & Cogburn, 1997
	Moos Work Environment Scale	Moos, 1994
	Work Organization Assessment Questionnaire	Griffiths, Cox, Karanika, Khan, & Tomas, 2006
	Work Organization Assessment Tool	Howard, Spielholz, Bao, Silverstein, & Fan, 2009
Performance Skills		
Motor and praxis skills: Functional capacity evaluation (FCE)	Blankenship FCE System	Brubaker et al., 2007
	Cal–FCP	Matheson, Mooney, Grant, Leggett, & Kenny, 1996
	ErgoScience Physical Work Performance Evaluation	Tuckwell, Straker, & Barrett, 2002
	Gibson Approach to FCE	Gibson, Strong, & Wallace, 2005

Table 3. Examples of Selected Assessments *(cont.)*

Area of Evaluation	Assessment	Reference
	Performance Skills *(cont.)*	
Motor and praxis skills: Functional capacity evaluation (FCE) *(cont.)*	Isernhagen/WorkWell System	Gross, Battié, & Cassidy, 2004
	Progressive Isoinertial Lifting Evaluation	Lygren, Dragesund, Joensen, Ask, & Moe-Nilssen, 2005
	WorkHab FCE	Legge & Burgess-Limerick, 2007
Motor and praxis skills: Other	EPIC Lift Test	Matheson, 1996
	Get-Up-and-Go Test	Mathias, Nayak, & Isaacs, 1986
	Minnesota Manual Dexterity Test	Gloss & Wardle, 1982
	Moberg Pickup Test	Ng, Ho, & Chow, 1999
	Upper Extremity Function Scale	Pransky, Feuerstein, Himmelstein, Katz, & Vickers-Lahti, 1997
	Valpar #9 Whole Body Range of Motion	Available from Valpar International (www.valparint.com/WS9.htm)
	Isometric testing (Chatillon force gauge) Job simulated testing	
Sensory–perceptual skills	Sensory testing (touch, temperature, pinprick, kinesthesia, proprioception, two-point discrimination, vibration) Visual acuity Color vision testing Visual field testing Hearing test Olfactory test Figure–ground test Depth perception	
Emotional regulation skills	Job-simulated testing Observation	
Cognitive skills	Behavioral Assessment of the Dysexecutive Syndrome	Wilson, Alderman, Burgess, Emslie, & Evans, 1996
	Bennett Hand–Tool Dexterity Test	Bennett, 1985
	Executive Function Performance Test	Baum, Morrison, Hahn, & Edwards, 2003, 2008
	Oral Directions Test	Field, Bayley, & Bayley, 1977
	Test of Everyday Attention	Robertson, Ward, Ridgeway, & Nimmo-Smith, 1996
	Wonderlic Personnel Test	Dodrill, 1983
Communication and social skills	Job-simulated testing Observation	
	Client Factors: Body Function	
Muscle strength	Grip strength testing Pinch strength testing	Mathiowetz et al., 1985

(continued)

Table 3. Examples of Selected Assessments *(cont.)*

Area of Evaluation	Assessment	Reference
	Client Factors: Body Function *(cont.)*	
Muscle strength *(cont.)*	Manual muscle testing Isometric strength testing Isotonic testing Isokinetic strength testing	
Range of motion, flexibility	Sit and reach test	American Alliance for Health, Physical Education, Recreation, and Dance, 1988 Prudential Fitnessgram, 1992
	Goniometry Inclinometry Clinical observation	
Muscle endurance	ACSM protocol	Whaley, Brubaker, & Otto, 2006
	YMCA tests	Golding, 2000
Coordination	Crawford Small Parts	Crawford & Crawford, 1956
	Minnesota Manual Dexterity Test	Gloss & Wardle, 1982 Lafayette Instrument
	Nine-Hole Peg Test	Kellor, Frost, Silberber, Iversen, & Cummings, 1971
	O'Connell Finger Dexterity Test	Fleishman & Hempel, 1954
	Purdue Pegboard	Tiffin, 1999
Balance	Berg Balance Scale	Berg, Wood-Dauphinee, & Williams, 1995
	Tinetti Balance Scale	Cipriany-Dacko, Innerst, Johannsen, & Rude, 1997
Posture	Clinical observation	
Gait	Clinical observation	
Stamina, fatigue, effort	Borg Perceived Exertion Scale	Borg, 1990
	Multidimensional Assessment of Fatigue Scale	Belza, Henke, Yelin, Epstein, & Gilliss, 1993
	Need for Recovery After Work	de Croon, Sluiter, & Frings-Dresen, 2003
	Talk Test	Persinger, Foster, Gibson, Fater, & Pocari, 2004
	YMCA Step Test	Golding, 2000
	Rockport Walking Test	Kline et al., 1987; Pober, Freedson, Kline, McKinnis, & Rippe, 2002
	Six-Minute Walk Test	American Thoracic Society, 2002; Solway, Brooks, Lacasse, & Thomas, 2001

Table 3. Examples of Selected Assessments *(cont.)*

Area of Evaluation	Assessment	Reference
	Client Factors: Body Function *(cont.)*	
Pain functions	Brief Pain Inventory	Ger, Ho, Sun, Wang, & Cleeland, 1999
	Dallas Pain Questionnaire	Lawlis, Cuencas, Selby, & McCoy, 1989
	Graded Chronic Pain Scale	Dworking et al., 2002
	Low Back Pain Rating Scale	Manniche et al., 1994
	McGill Pain Questionnaire	Melzack, 1975
	Pain Catastrophizing Scale	Vlaeyen, Kole-Snijders, Boeren, & Van Eek, 1995
	Pain Disability Index	Tait, Pollard, Margolis, Duckro, & Krause, 1987
	Pain Self-Efficacy Questionnaire	Nicholas, 1994
	Ransford Pain Diagram	Ohnmeiss, Vanharanta, & Elholm, 1999
	University of Alabama Pain Behavior Scale	Feldt, 2000
	Pain diagram 0–10 pain rating scale Visual analogue scale	
Mental functions	Awareness Questionnaire	Sherer, Bergloff, Boake, High, & Levin, 1998
	Fear Avoidance Beliefs Questionnaire	Waddel, Newton, Henderson, Somerville, & Main, 1003
	Gage Self-Efficacy Scale	Gage, Noh, Polatajko, & Kasper, 1994
	Hamilton Anxiety Scale	Hamilton, 1969
	Hopkin's Symptom State Anxiety Score of the Spielberger State–Anxiety Inventory, Checklist	Derogatis, 1977
	Center for Epidemiological Studies–Depression	Radloff, 1977
	Beck Depression Inventory	Beck, Ward, Mendelson, Mock, & Erbaugh,1961; Beck, Rial, & Rickets,1974
	Life Stressors and Social Resources Inventory	Moos, 1988
	Patient Competency Rating Scale	Prigatano, Altman, & O'Brien, 1990
	Self-Awareness of Deficits Interview	Sherer et al., 1998
	Test of Everyday Attention	Robertson, Ward, Ridgeway, & Nimmo-Smith, 1996
	Job-simulated testing Clinical observation	

(continued)

Table 3. Examples of Selected Assessments (cont.)

Area of Evaluation	Assessment	Reference
Client Factors: Body Function (cont.)		
Sensation and nerve function	Light touch Sharp–dull discrimination Temperature discrimination Proprioception Kinesthesia Static and moving two-point discrimination Semmes–Weinstein monofilaments Vibrometry threshold tests Snellen visual acuity Visual field testing Eye dominance testing Visual scanning Lighthouse Near Visual Acuity Test Clinical observation of functional hearing Scratch-and-sniff job-related smell identification	
Client Factors: Body Structures		
Circulation and oxygenation	Blood pressure Heart rate Respiration rate Oxygen saturation Allen's test	
Body composition	Body weight Body mass index	
Skin and wound integrity	Clinical observation of wounds, cuts, abrasions, and skin integrity	
Muscle integrity	Muscle length testing Modified Ashworth Scale (spasticity) Drop arm test Palpation	Ashworth, 1964
Joint structural integrity	Ligament testing Grind test Joint capsule length testing Accessory joint motions	
Nerve integrity	Tinel's sign Phalen test Provocative testing	

reliability (Reneman, Fokkens, Dijkstra, Geertzen, & Groothoff, 2005), test–retest reliability (Reneman et al., 2004), predictive validity (Gross et al., 2004), and construct validity (Gross & Battié, 2003). A 2-day assessment allows the therapist to monitor the client's response to the first day of testing and determine if that effort can be sustained on back-to-back days. However, a second day of testing was not found to be necessary when using the Isernhagen/WorkWell System (Reneman, Dijkstra, Westmaas, & Göeken, 2002).

Research has also established the reliability and/or validity of the California Functional Capacity Protocol (Matheson, 1996), the ErgoScience Physical Work Performance Evaluation (Tuckwell, Straker, & Barrett, 2002), the JobFit System based on the WorkHab FCE (Legge & Burgess-Limerick, 2007), the Gibson Approach to Functional Capacity Evaluation for chronic back pain clients (Gibson, Strong, & Wallace, 2005), the Blankenship FCE (Brubaker et al., 2007), the EPIC Lift Capacity Test (Jay et al., 2000), and the Progressive Isoinertial Lifting Evaluation (Lygren et al., 2005). Many FCE protocols or lift capacity tests require the therapist to participate in training and/or certification to ensure standardization and adherence to test procedures.

Role of Pain in the Work Assessment Evaluation

Clients referred for an occupational therapy work evaluation may be experiencing residual pain from the damaged body structures or the resultant limitations. *Pain* is a complex phenomenon that involves "psychological arousal, sensations of noxious stimulation, tissue damage or irritation, behavioral avoidance, complaints of subjective distress, and the social environment" (Engel, 2006, p. 649). The presence of pain does not mean that a client cannot work; however, pain can distract the client's focus from the job duties and affect job safety and performance.

The occupational therapist seeks to understand the client's pain and its effect on performance. A client who is fearful that his or her pain may result in additional trauma will be hesitant to perform tasks while symptomatic. Conversely, a client who believes in "no pain, no gain" may be overly aggressive during the work evaluation. Therefore, the occupational therapist questions the client about his or her pain, including the factors that increase it, strategies that help manage it, and its effect on daily living. Throughout the work evaluation, the therapist uses instruments to measure the client's pain and observes the client's pain-related behaviors and ability to manage symptoms. By forming a therapeutic relationship with the client and gaining an understanding of the client's pain-related behaviors and management strategies, the therapist can make appropriate decisions regarding the progression of the work evaluation.

If the client is taking medication to manage pain, the occupational therapist usually instructs the client to take the medication as prescribed during the evaluation. If the medication affects a client's ability to drive or operate machinery, the therapist takes this into consideration when making return-to-work recommendations. Some pain medications can affect a client's mood, energy, cognition (e.g., concentration, processing speed), sensory functions (e.g., vision, balance), or motor functions (e.g., coordination, speed of movement). Therefore, the therapist proceeds with testing in line with the findings of the safety screen. If the client will not be allowed to work on the current medication regimen, it is best for the physician to wean the client off the medication before the evaluation so that the therapist can accurately appraise the client's capacity to work.

Evaluation Outcomes

A critical step in the occupational therapy evaluation process is the synthesis of the assessment results. The occupational therapist writes an evaluation report summarizing the results of the evaluation and making recommendations for future care. If treatment is indicated, the report includes a comprehensive intervention plan. If the evaluation is to determine if the client is able to return to work, the report compares the client's performance and results of the various assessments with the activity demands of the job and the contextual requirements of the work environment and makes recommendations regarding the client's return to work. If modifications to the work tasks, equipment or tools, or environment are needed to support the client's return to work, the evaluation report identifies them. If the client lacks the capacity to return to the job and the therapist believes that the client has the potential to return to work following occupational therapy intervention, the report recommends continued treatment and estimates rehabilitation potential. The evaluation report identifies areas that support and limit performance and problems related to the client's occupations, particularly work performance, but also performance in other daily activities and occupations such as self-care, home management, and leisure, which may have an effect on work performance.

For example, on examination, a client referred to occupational therapy for carpal tunnel syndrome may demonstrate a positive Tinel's sign suggesting entrapment of the nerve (body structure), lack of discriminative sensation in the thumb and index finger (body structures), impaired fine motor coordination and manipulation skills (body functions), poor forearm positioning of the wrists rested on the edge of the desk during typing activity (performance patterns), impaired accuracy after typing for 20 minutes, and numbness with prolonged mouse use (performance skills). However, the client's strengths may include good compliance with splint wearing, willingness to change her habits, and the employer's interest in exploring voice recognition software. Limitations identified may include the client's obesity and the noise level at her workstation, which may affect the ability to use voice recognition software. Occupational performance issues may be that her leisure, work, and household activities all involve repetitive manipulations that are placing her at risk of continued symptoms.

Intervention

Intervention Plan

As part of the occupational therapy process, the occupational therapist develops an intervention plan that documents the client's return-to-work goals, the treatment approaches, and recommendations or referrals to other professionals if indicated. The plan outlines and guides the therapist's actions and is based on selected theories and frames of reference and the best available evidence to meet the identified outcomes (AOTA, 2008b).

The intervention plan includes different components depending on the results of the evaluation, the client's goals, the client's health status, and contextual factors. The plan for an individual who has an acute hand injury that requires daily wound management and range-of-motion (ROM) exercises will involve intricate steps to enhance healing and restore function

of the hand. An individual who displays the capacity to work during the initial evaluation may need only one therapy session to learn how to prevent future problems from occurring. Another client who has sustained a work-related brain injury may have a comprehensive rehabilitation plan to restore or learn compensatory strategies for impaired cognition.

The plan for the client with carpal tunnel syndrome may be to identify the risk factors that contribute to her condition, to competently use voice activation software to prepare electronic documents in the occupational therapy clinic, and to perform tendon-gliding exercises twice daily. Long-term goals may be to consistently maintain good typing posture, to use a computer mouse with her non-affected hand, to follow a balanced schedule of hand use for work and home activities, and to effectively use strategies to compensate for hand numbness and weakness.

In the intervention plan, the occupational therapist identifies intervention approaches to be used, as well as specific short- and long-term treatment goals. The long-term goals reflect functional levels of performance for the various occupations required for the client's specific situation. Goals included in the plan are specific and measurable, including the level of performance and time frame for achievement. The goals of treatment may vary during different phases of recovery. Initially treatment may focus on protecting the surgically repaired structures from damage by fabricating a splint, elevating the injured hand to combat edema, and teaching the client how to perform daily tasks without using the injured hand (including both work-related and non-work-related tasks). As healing occurs treatment may focus on restoration of the function of these structures, such as the ability of the tendon to glide and the joint to move through ROM. Use of the injured hand to manipulate objects and perform work tasks is performed after the structures are strong enough to tolerate external forces. However, a client may be capable of returning to work with compensations at any point in recovery in which it is felt that he or she can safely perform job tasks without posing risk of injury to himself or herself or others.

Intervention Implementation

Treatment begins soon after the initial evaluation. The frequency of sessions varies, depending on the physician's orders, the occupational therapist's recommendations, and the client's situation, but usually ranges from daily to once or twice per month. The frequency of treatment may or may not be associated with the phase of recovery. For example, an individual who just underwent a tenolysis procedure to free up a previously repaired tendon that has become adhered may need the occupational therapist to assist with tendon gliding exercises twice daily. However, once the client or caregiver learns how to perform these interventions independently, occupational therapy may decrease to once weekly. In other cases, the frequency of treatment may increase. For example, a client participating in a weekly occupational therapy program for strengthening may advance to daily sessions when a more aggressive program is appropriate. The duration of the treatment session may also vary; session length may increase from weekly 30-min outpatient therapy visits to 3- to 8-hr work hardening sessions.

Factors that influence the intervention plan include the client's current and previous occupations, diagnosis, acuteness or chronicity of the condition, previous and current medical history, age, fitness level, other treatments (e.g., medication, surgery, therapy), availability for treatment, setting, preferences, physician's orders, compliance and follow-through, pain tolerance, and self-limiting behavior. The client's comorbid conditions can provide additional challenges during the rehabilitation process; hypertension, cardiac conditions, and pulmonary conditions require close monitoring by the occupational therapist. Intervention for the primary referral diagnosis may place stress on the cardiopulmonary system, so the occupational therapist may need to modify assessment and intervention methods or use a different treatment approach. The occupational therapist always places the safety of the client first; therefore, rehabilitation

may need to occur at a slower pace or using modified techniques.

Occupational therapy practitioners tailor intervention approaches to enable clients to meet their goals. The intervention approaches used may vary during the course of treatment and from client to client. Because the long-term goal of occupational therapy is to improve the client's occupational performance, the therapist uses the approaches that best match the client's needs. Occupational therapy intervention approaches, typically used in combination, include the following:

- *Create* or *promote* occupational performance
- *Establish* or *restore* occupational performance
- *Maintain* occupational performance
- *Modify* occupational performance
- *Prevent* deterioration of occupational performance.

Examples of occupational therapy interventions under the rubric of these five approaches as outlined in the *Framework* are provided in Table 4. The occupational therapist considers the types of interventions available when determining the most effective treatment plan for a given client. The types of interventions include therapeutic use of self; therapeutic use of occupations and activities, which include occupation-based interventions, purposeful activity, and preparatory methods; consultation; advocacy; and education.

Use of the entire range of intervention approaches for a client with a work-related injury can be very effective. In using the prevention approach with a client who has early symptoms, the occupational therapy practitioner teaches the client methods to perform work tasks that will decrease exposure to harmful postures, forces, and work methods to allow for healing of the structures; develops a stretching or strengthening program to condition the structures for the work task; or modifies the work environment to decrease the exposure. The following sections describe these approaches in more detail and provide examples of occupational therapy interventions for work rehabilitation.

Table 4. Intervention Approaches and Examples of Occupation-Based Goals for Clients With Work-Related Injuries

Approach	Focus of Intervention	Examples of Occupation-Based Goals
Restore/remediate: Designed to change client variables to establish a skill or ability that has been impaired (Dunn, McClain, Brown, & Youngstrom, 1998)	Body structures	Perform tendon-gliding exercises to allow finger to tightly grasp gun trigger
	Body functions	Perform finger tapping quickly and accurately to prepare to type
	Performance skills	Lift 50-lb box from floor to waist
	Performance patterns	Establish appropriate rest–work cycle during assembly line work
	Occupation	Accurately type monthly report
Modify, compensate, adapt: Designed to find ways to revise the task, method, or environment to support performance (Dunn et al., 1998)	Body functions	Use jar opener to compensate for grip loss on the job
	Performance skills	Use scooter for mobility from the parking lot
	Occupation	Use voice activation software for word processing
	Context	Lower desk height to avoid bending during pipette task
	Activity demands	Reduce the weight of the load lifted overhead
Maintain: Designed to provide the supports that will preserve the performance capabilities clients have regained so they can continue to meet their occupational needs	Body functions	Perform exercise program to maintain fitness level for work
	Performance skills	Use proper body mechanics while transferring patients
	Context	Maintain clear walkways in work area to avoid falls while carrying
	Performance patterns	Develop habit of wearing back brace when handling heavy loads
Prevent: Designed to prevent performance problems by supporting body structures and functions, performance skills, environment, and habits and routines (Dunn et al., 1998)	Performance patterns	Perform stretch before work shift and hourly throughout work day
	Context	Use sit/stand workstation for typing tasks
	Body functions	Use overhead lift to perform all lifting tasks
	Activity demands	Decrease number of repetitions required on assembly line
Create/promote: Does not assume a disability is present or any factors interfere with performance; designed to provide enriched contextual and activity experiences that enhance performance for all persons in the natural contexts of life (Dunn et al., 1998)	Context	Design barrier-free workplace
	Body functions	Establish on-site wellness programs to promote fitness
	Activity demands	Use assistive technology to eliminate manual material handling on the job

Create or Promote Occupational Performance

The create or promote approach removes the focus from a disability or other factors interfering with performance. Occupational therapists using this approach provide enriched contextual and activity experiences that will enhance the performance of all persons in the natural contexts of life (Dunn et al., 1998). For example, an employer may ask an occupational therapist to evaluate a workstation and make ergonomic changes to ensure that employ-ees are performing tasks safely. Because occupational therapists are experts at analyzing tasks, an employer may ask a therapist to measure the demands of a job and design a postoffer, preplacement screening to ensure that new hires are able to perform the essential functions of the job safely and competitively. An employer may also ask the therapist to participate on an ergonomic team, conduct educational sessions, or provide other types of on-site services to enhance the comfort of the entire workforce. This approach promotes the safety and health of all individuals in the workplace and helps prevent work-related illnesses and injuries.

Establish or Restore Occupational Performance

The establish or restore approach is directed at restoring or remediating function that approximates levels before the onset of the disease or deterioration. Strategies are focused entirely on the person and are geared toward building skills or remediating deficits (Dunn Brown, & McGuigan, 1994). This approach uses occupation as the end result and places emphasis on restoration of performance skills, performance patterns, and client factors. The possibilities for remediation are not absolute for all skills, and the occupational therapist must consider the type and cause of each deficit area before attempting remediation. If the client's limited functional capacities prevent safe work performance, the therapist may use the restorative approach—for example, by fabricating a dynamic hand splint to improve mobility, training the client to use a computerized work simulator to increase grip strength and hand use, or participating in a daily work hardening program to build the client's tolerance for tool use and improve lifting capacities. Establishing safe work habits and routines—for example, through postural training or education in proper tool use—are also an emphasis of this approach.

Maintain Occupational Performance

The maintain approach is used in occupational therapy intervention to provide supports that will allow clients to preserve their performance capabilities and prevent deterioration of function. The occupational therapist helps the client with a work-related injury maintain the function of the noninjured body parts and systems. A client who sustained a hand injury may benefit from shoulder ROM exercises to maintain flexibility and a walking program to maintain cardiovascular health. Once function of the injured body part or system has been restored, the therapist may design a program to maintain the gains made during treatment. The maintenance approach may help to prevent further work-related injuries or illnesses.

Modify Occupational Performance

The modify approach adapts current circumstances to facilitate occupational performance. This approach does not attempt to restore the client's func-tion to premorbid levels but rather aims to facilitate optimal engagement at the current level of function. When the client does not demonstrate the work capacities to perform the job, modifications can be made to the client's approach or methods of work performance or the work environment or context the task occurs within, or the demands of the work task may be modified to

allow the client to return to work (Dunn et al., 1994, 1998).

To prevent interruption in occupational performance, the occupational therapist may use a compensatory approach early in rehabilitation. For example, the therapist teaches an individual whose hand is immobilized how to perform tasks such as driving, cooking, and typing with one hand or shows a client who is not able to bend how to lift objects from the floor or put on shoes independently. A preventive approach may complement this compensatory approach when, for example, the occupational therapist instructs the client who is able to use only one hand to take rest breaks to avoid overuse of the noninjured hand or teaches methods to avoid injuring the back when lifting.

A compensatory approach is also frequently used when a client has permanent impairments that cannot be restored. For example, a client who uses a prosthetic hook after losing a hand at work may need tools adapted to couple with the prosthesis or automated methods to perform a work task. For another client who now must sit to work and cannot reach to high or low surfaces, the occupational therapist may help the employer modify the work surface heights so the client can still perform the work tasks independently. All of these modifications require the client to learn new ways to perform the job.

In addition to modifying the task, the method of engaging in the task, or the environment, the occupational therapist commonly provides education about these modifications. The therapist explains modified techniques to the client, discussing such concepts as body mechanics, work–rest cycles, stretches or brief pauses in work that allow muscles to stretch or rest, and other methods to compensate for their work-related injury or illness.

Context

Modifying contextual factors results in improved performance by altering the environment to better match the person's skills and abilities. The modify strategy promotes a more supportive context to improve performance. The employer must be actively engaged if the work environment requires modification. Modifications to the workstation may be easy to make, such as lowering a desk or increasing the lighting in a work cubicle, but changing the larger context may be more difficult, such as shifting a nurse with a work-related injury to a unit where the clients are less acute so the lifting demands are decreased or having a carpenter who cannot climb stay on the ground and prepare wood for the other carpenters to install from ladders and scaffolds.

Activity Demands

Modifying a task's activity demands to match the person's skills and abilities can result in improved task performance. Occupational therapists combine their skills in activity analysis with their ability to evaluate the client's ability to perform the task to make activity demand modifications that promote work performance. Components of the task that exceed the client's current capacities may be modified so the client can successfully perform the task; examples include reorganizing the work so a client can perform a portion of the task that is within his or her capacity, slowing the pace the client must maintain, or allowing the client to rotate through a variety of work tasks to decrease his or her exposure to tasks that are problematic.

Equipment or tools may be used to modify the activity demands. The client may need to use a different type of tool that will make the task easier, such as a smaller floor mop or a roller-ball mouse, or adaptive equipment may be fabricated to improve task performance, such as a splint to modify the grasp on a pen or the addition of handles to a container that the client must manipulate. The employer may choose to make these activity demand modifications a requirement for the client, a step otherwise referred to as an *administrative control*.

Prevent Deterioration of Occupational Performance

Occupational therapy intervention can also prevent acceleration in the deterioration of function. Although preventing disease progression is outside the domain of occupational therapy, preventing or slowing deterioration in occupational performance is a unique contribution of occupational therapy intervention. This outcome is achieved through provision of adaptive methods or equipment; environmental support; modification of habits and routines; and education of the client, coworkers, family, and employer. Empowering the client to use and build on strategies already in place will assist in preserving work performance. For example, the occupational therapist may help the client identify nonadaptive work methods or environments, brainstorm alternatives, and collaborate with coworkers and management to implement changes.

Clients must learn to problem solve and self-manage on a day-to-day basis to prevent and manage work performance problems. Teaching clients these skills may help them avoid exacerbating the condition from which they are recuperating or other conditions that may arise due to overuse. For example, a client who must use a wheelchair while recuperating from bilateral leg injuries may develop tendonitis in the shoulder from pushing the wheelchair. Provision of a closer parking space to limit wheelchair pushing, instruction in proper wheelchair propulsion method, and use of rest breaks may help to prevent exacerbation of this condition.

Intervention Review

Intervention review is a continuous process of reevaluating and reviewing the intervention plan, the effectiveness of service delivery, and progress toward targeted outcomes (AOTA, 2008b). Reevaluation may involve readministering assessments or tests that were used at the time of initial evaluation, having the client complete a satisfaction questionnaire, or answering questions to evaluate each goal. Reevaluation substantiates progress toward goal attainment; indicates any change in functional status; and directs modifications to the intervention plan, if necessary (Moyers & Dale, 2007).

When treating a client who is unable to work and is receiving workers' compensation benefits, the occupational therapist regularly reviews the client's progress and determines if return to work is safe and feasible.

If it becomes apparent during the intervention review that the client can perform portions of his or her job, the therapist informs the physician, case manager, and/or employer of the duties that can and cannot be performed and the task, work schedule, or environmental modifications that are necessary to support return to work. At times, a client can return to modified work within his or her capacities while continuing with rehabilitation to maximize tolerances in preparation for regular work duties.

Documentation

Occupational therapy practitioners carefully document their services in the areas of evaluation, intervention, and outcomes (AOTA, 2008a). For clients with work-related injuries or illnesses, practitioners document their recommendations related to work limitations and communicate them to the employer, physician, and other team members. This documentation should be completed "within the time frames, format, and standards established by the practice settings, agencies, external accreditation programs, payers and AOTA documents" (AOTA, 2005, p. 664).

"The purpose of occupational therapy documentation is to
1. Articulate the rationale for the provision of occupational therapy services and the relationship of this service to the client's outcomes
2. Reflect the therapist's clinical reasoning and professional judgment
3. Communicate information about the client from an occupational therapy perspective
4. Create a chronological record of client status, occupational therapy services provided, and client outcomes" (AOTA, 2008a p. 684).

The following types of documentation may be completed for each client, as required by legal requirements, the practice setting, third-party payers, or some combination of these:
- Evaluation or screening report (including functional capacity evaluation report)
- Occupational therapy service contacts
- Occupational therapy intervention plan
- Progress report
- Prescription or recommendation for adaptive equipment
- Reevaluation report
- Discharge or discontinuation report (AOTA, 2008a).

Functional capacity evaluation reports should follow the recommendations of the Functional Assessment Network (2003) to support a collaborative process for return-to-work planning and disability management. Documentation must disclose all sources of information that were used to formulate the conclusions (assessment tools, methods, observations, worker's perceptions, and feedback); clearly describe the match between the worker's abilities and the job criteria and work environment; and provide conclusions that identify the worker's abilities, limitations, and barriers in terms of return to work, with each conclusion supported by a rationale that flows logically from the findings (Functional Assessment Network, 2003). The "Guidelines for Documentation of Occupational Therapy" (AOTA, 2008a) outline specific report contents and fundamental elements of documentation.

Discharge and Discontinuation Planning

Planning for discharge begins with the initial evaluation and continues during each subsequent visit. The occupational therapist must have a thorough understanding of the job duties and the work environment before recommending return to work. If the therapist determines that there is a match between the client's work capacities and the work requirements, he or she initiates the return-to-work process, which may require modifications in the work duties, work schedule, and work environment or the use of devices or equipment the client needs to return to work. The occupational therapist documents these recommendations and describes current work capacities in the discharge or discontinuation report. If the client is still progressing in occupational therapy and continued treatment is indicated even though the client is returning to work, the report recommends continuation of care. If a client stops making progress in treatment or has reached a plateau, the report recommends discontinuation of treatment. At the time of discharge from services, some clients still do not demonstrate the capacity to return to work. In the discharge or discontinuation report, the occupational therapist outlines the client's present work capacity so that he or she can move on to the next phase of the process, be it disability determination, vocational rehabilitation, retirement, or other medical procedures.

Outcomes and Follow-Up

Potential outcomes of an occupational therapy program designed to facilitate the return to work include the client's return to his or her previous job on a full-time basis, return to the job with modified work duties or work schedule or light-duty work, transfer to a new job, or remaining off work. The occupational therapy practitioner follows up with clients who have returned to full-duty or modified work. Ongoing consultation with the employer may be needed to monitor the worker's response to the work duties and environment, to identify additional adjustments to the work modifications to best match the client's current capacities and prevent future injuries, and to recommend the resumption of full work duties when appropriate.

After the client is discharged from occupational therapy services, additional intervention may be needed at a later date. This need may arise if the client experiences a decline in health, an exacerbation of a previous condition, recovery from an intervening medical condition, a medical intervention that alters the client's ability to work, age-related changes, or a change in the work context. Any of these factors may prompt the employer or client to request on-site consultation to help the client maintain work performance and prevent subsequent injuries or illnesses. Therapists therefore may maintain an open relationship with the client and his or her employer after discharge so these clients feel comfortable seeking assistance for additional intervention when necessary.

■ ■ ■

Intervention: Evidence-Based Literature Review

This section summarizes the results of four systematic reviews of the scientific literature related to occupational therapy interventions for individuals with injuries and/or illnesses commonly sustained on the job. The reviews were based on four focused questions derived from specific areas of practice—low back; elbow; forearm, wrist, and hand; and shoulder. The reviews include studies from the occupational therapy literature and related fields describing interventions that are within the scope of occupational therapy.

The section responding to each question begins with background information related to the focus area, provides an overview of the role of occupational therapy in that area, states the literature review question, synthesizes the results of the review, and closes with a summary of key findings from the research literature. The final section discusses implications of the systematic literature review and provides recommendations for occupational therapy practice that incorporate the evidence from the review with suggestions from content experts in occupational therapy and work and industry. Appendix A provides background information related to the evidence-based literature review and a complete summary of the methodology used for the systematic reviews and the recommendation process.

Question 1. Interventions to the Low Back

According to the U.S. Bureau of Labor Statistics (BLS; 2008), musculoskeletal disorders accounted for 29% of injuries and illnesses requiring days away from work in 2007. The part of the body most affected by work-related incidents was the trunk (including the shoulder and back), accounting for 33% of all cases. Injuries and illnesses to the back constituted 62% of the days-away-from-work cases involving the trunk. Furthermore, low back pain is estimated to affect 80% of the world's population (WHO, 2003). The most common work-related conditions of the low back include herniated intervertebral discs, sacroiliitis, radicular pain syndromes (including sciatica), muscle strains, ligament sprains, nonspecific low back pain, and lumbar radiculopathy.

Occupational therapy practitioners perform client-centered evaluations and direct clients with low back injuries in the performance of occupations and activities using a variety of approaches, including instruction in proper body mechanics and ways to perform activities safely; task analysis and use of ergonomic design to modify the environment; use of relaxation techniques, work hardening, and reconditioning; and education for pain management, stress reduction, and coping (Grangaard, 2006; Maher & Bear-Lehman, 2008).

The evidence-based literature review question asked, "What occupational therapy interventions are effective in the rehabilitation of individuals with work-related low back injuries and illnesses?" The studies in this review include seven that examined the effects of therapeutic exercise; two that focused on client education; four that investigated activity, functional restoration, or work reconditioning; two that investigated the effect of physical agent modalities; four that examined cognitive–behavioral-oriented approaches; and five that evaluated multidisciplinary or biopsychosocial approaches (some studies are included in more than one category).

This review of the evidence revealed that effective interventions directed at clients with low back injury or illness share some common features. The evidence is insufficient to support or refute the effectiveness of exercise therapy and other conservative treatments for subacute and chronic low back injuries. No significant difference was found in short-term pain relief between exercise therapy and no treatment for acute low back injuries. Likewise, there was no difference in pain relief with exercise therapy compared with other conservative treatments; exercise therapy did not have a significant effect on functional outcomes for acute low back injuries.

The evidence does, however, support a biopsychosocial approach to work-related low back rehabilitation with the following key features:

- Therapist-directed and supervised therapeutic exercises targeting the individual client's symptoms (stretching, ROM, flexibility, endurance, and strengthening)
- Client education (proper body mechanics, back education)
- Graded functional activity (work reconditioning, on-site interventions, graduated return to work)
- Environmental modifications (work site visit, ergonomic modifications)
- Cognitive–behavioral strategies (positive reinforcement, progressive relaxation, biofeedback)
- Multidisciplinary approach.

The following paragraphs summarize the key findings.

Filiz, Cakmak, and Ozcan (2005) compared two exercise programs with a control condition following lumbar disc surgery in a Level I randomized controlled study. Sixty participants who had had a lumbar disc operation (single-level discectomy) for the first time were randomly assigned to three groups. The first group received an intensive exercise program and back-school education, and the second group received a home exercise program and back-school education. The third group was the control group and did not receive education or exercise training. Participants treated with intensive exercise and back-school education experienced a significant decrease in severity of pain and disability, and they returned to work or daily activities after surgery significantly sooner than the other two groups. The group that received a home exercise program and back-school education returned to work and/or daily activities significantly sooner than the control group. Both exercise groups had significantly better results than the control group for perceived low back disability. Only the intensive exercise group had better results than the control group on self-reported depression inventory. This study was limited by lack of long-term follow-up and a relatively small number of participants.

In a Level I randomized controlled trial, Koumantakis, Watson, and Oldham (2005) examined the usefulness of the addition of specific stabilization exercises to a general back and abdominal muscle exercise approach for 55 patients with subacute or chronic nonspecific back pain. They compared a specific muscle stabilization–enhanced general exercise approach with a general exercise–only approach. Group 1 participated in an exercise program that focused on the flexor and extensor muscle group. Group 2 participated in a stabilizing exercise program that focused on stabilizing postural muscles. Both groups showed improvement following intervention. Perceived disability was significantly lower for the general exercise–only group immediately posttreatment, but this difference was no longer present at 3-month follow-up. For all remaining outcome measures (pain, locus of control, fear, self-efficacy), both groups improved immediately following intervention, and these improvements were maintained 3 months later. No between-group differences were detected at either time. This study was limited by a small sample size.

Hurwitz, Morgenstern, and Chiao (2005) examined the effectiveness of recreational physical activity and back exercises on low back pain, related disability, and psychological distress. The authors used a Level I randomized controlled trial that included 681 participants divided into four groups: Group 1 received chiropractic care with physical modalities, Group 2 received chiropractic care without physical modalities, Group 3 received medical care with physical therapy, and Group 4 received medical care without physical therapy. The authors found moderate evidence that flexion exercises are not effective in reducing acute pain, strong evidence that extension exercises are not effective in reducing acute pain, no evidence that flexion exercises are effective in reducing chronic pain, no evidence that strengthening exercises are effective in reducing acute pain, and strong evidence that strengthening exercises are not more effective than other types of exercise. Thus, specific back exercises may be counterproductive, and restoration of normal functioning should instead be emphasized. Because participants were primary care patients, they may not be representative of individuals with low back pain in clinical settings (i.e., those receiving workers' compensation may differ) or those who do not seek clinical treatment at all. In addition, the authors did not collect information on specific types of back exercises; they relied on participants' self-reports.

In a Level I systematic review, Heymans, van Tulder, Esmail, Bombardier, and Koes (2004) sought to determine if back schools were more effective than other treatments or no treatment for patients with recurrent and chronic, nonspecific low back pain. Their review included 19 studies with a total of 3,584 patients. The authors were unable to identify strong evidence for any particular type of back-school treatment. They found moderate evidence that back schools had better short- and intermediate-term effects than other treatments for recurrent and chronic low back pain in terms of pain level and functional status. There was moderate evidence that back schools in a work setting are more effective than other treatments, placebo, or waiting list controls in improving functional status and promoting return to work during short- and intermediate-term follow-up. Randomized controlled trials included in this review were overall of low methodological quality, characterized by lack of blinding of patients, observers, and care providers; inappropriate methods of randomization; inadequate concealment of treatment allocation; and the presence of cointerventions.

Hagen, Hilde, Jamtvedt, and Winnem (2004) conducted a Level I systematic review to assess the effects of advice to rest in bed for patients with acute low back pain or sciatica. They reviewed 11 trials involving 1,963 patients. Persons with low back pain who were advised to rest in bed had slightly more pain and less functional recovery than those advised to stay active. For patients with sciatica, there was strong evidence of little or no difference in pain or functional status between bed rest and staying active. For patients with acute low back pain, there was moderate evidence of little or no difference in pain intensity or functional status between bed rest and exercises. For patients with sciatica, there was moderate evidence of little or no difference in pain intensity between bed rest and physical therapy, but there were small improvements in functional status with physical therapy. There was moderate evidence of little or no difference in pain intensity or functional status between 2 to 3 days of rest and 7 days of rest.

A Level I randomized controlled trial by Staal et al. (2004) sought to determine the effectiveness of a behavior-oriented graded activity program compared with usual care. The study included 134 participants who were workers absent from work because of low back pain. Participants were assigned to either graded activity (physical exercise, application of operant conditioning behavioral principles) or usual care (guidance and advice from an occupational physician, treatment by various caregivers). The authors found that graded activity for low back pain in an occupational health setting had a statistically significant effect on absence from work. The median days absent from work because of low back pain was 58 in the graded activity group and 87 in the usual care group. Functional status results showed a tendency toward improvement with graded activity that did not reach statistical significance. Interventions did not have a statistically significant impact on pain severity.

Schonstein, Kenny, Keating, and Koes (2003) conducted a Level I systematic review of randomized controlled trials to compare the effectiveness of physical conditioning programs such as work conditioning, work hardening, and functional restoration with that of management strategies that did not include traditional physical conditioning programs for workers with back and neck pain. They examined whether these programs differentially reduced time lost from work and increased functional status. The authors reviewed 18 randomized controlled trials; participants were adults who experienced disability at work because of back or neck pain. The review found that physical conditioning programs that included a cognitive–behavioral approach reduced the number of sick days lost at 12-month follow-up by an average of 45 days compared with general practitioner usual care for workers with chronic back pain. The review found insufficient evidence for or against the effectiveness of specific exercises that are not accompanied by a cognitive–behavioral approach in reducing sick days lost due to back pain for workers with either acute or chronic back pain.

Guzman et al. (2001) assessed the effect of multidisciplinary biopsychosocial rehabilitation on outcomes in patients with chronic low back pain in a Level I systematic review of 10 randomized controlled trials with a total of 1,964 participants. The authors found strong evidence that intensive (>100 hours of therapy) multidisciplinary biopsychosocial rehabilitation with functional restoration reduced pain and improved function in patients with chronic low back pain when compared with inpatient or outpatient nonmultidisciplinary treatments. They also found moderate evidence that intensive multidisciplinary biopsychosocial rehabilitation with functional restoration reduced pain when compared with outpatient nonmultidisciplinary rehabilitation or usual care. The evidence regarding vocational outcomes was contradictory; some trials reported improvement in work readiness with biopsychosocial rehabilitation, whereas others demonstrated no significant reduction in absenteeism. Less intensive interventions were not associated with improvements in clinically relevant outcomes.

In a systematic review and meta-analysis of randomized controlled trials of cognitive–behavioral therapy and behavior therapy for chronic pain, Morley, Eccleston, and Williams (1998) examined 25 trials that included 1,672 participants. Thirty-six percent were labeled as having chronic low back pain; 20% as having rheumatoid arthritis; 16% as having mixed, predominantly back pain; 8% as having osteoarthritis;

8% as having upper limb pain; 4% as having fibromyalgia; and 8% as having an unspecified condition. Compared with the waiting list control conditions, cognitive–behavioral treatments were associated with significant effect sizes on all domains of measurement. Comparison with alternative active treatments revealed that cognitive–behavioral treatments produced significantly greater changes for the domains of pain experience, cognitive coping and appraisal, and reduced behavioral expression of pain. The authors concluded that active psychological treatments based on the principle of cognitive–behavioral therapy are effective.

A pilot randomized controlled study involving 33 participants with chronic pain investigated the effect of work rehabilitation on improvement in the ability to work (Meyer, Fransen, Huwiler, Uebelhart, & Klipstein, 2005). The treatment group received interdisciplinary work rehabilitation, including work-specific exercises and education, that lasted for 8 weeks, 3.5 hr per day each working day. The control treatment took place with the allocating physician, who provided participants with specific recommendations concerning work reintegration, medication, and training. The results revealed no significant difference between the groups immediately posttreatment, but ability to work improved significantly at 8 weeks for both groups.

A Level I systematic review by Karjalainen et al. (2001) explored the effectiveness of multidisciplinary rehabilitation for subacute low back pain (more than 4 weeks but less than 3 months) for working-age adults whose back pain was not related to acute trauma, neoplasms, or inflammatory or neurological diseases. The authors included only multidisciplinary inpatient or outpatient programs (i.e., physician's consultation plus a psychological, social, or vocational intervention or a combination of these) and excluded trials consisting solely of medical treatment and physical therapy. They found only two relevant randomized, controlled trials for their review. These studies showed a statistically significant difference in return to work, with patients returning to work sooner in the intervention groups. Significant improvements were found in subjective disability and disorder-specific functional status for the intervention groups. No effects on intensity of pain could be attributed to the intervention. According to the authors, the methodological quality of the two trials was low; methodological defects included lack of blinding of patients, therapists, and observers and failure to report the effect of cointerventions.

Question 2. Interventions to the Elbow

Upper-extremity musculoskeletal disorders are often associated with repetitive and forceful work combined with awkward postures (i.e., excessive elbow flexion and/or supination and pronation). The BLS (2008) reported 54,260 cases of injuries to the arm (which includes the upper arm, elbow, and forearm) that required days away from work in 2007. This statistic represents 4.6% of the total number of nonfatal occupational injuries and illnesses involving days away from work reported in 2007.

The most common work-related elbow disorders include lateral epicondylitis, also known as "tennis elbow"; medial epicondylitis, also known as "golfer's elbow"; radial tunnel syndrome; and cubital tunnel syndrome.

Occupational therapy practitioners use a variety of interventions to relieve symptoms and facilitate the client's safe return to work. Interventions include ROM exercises, stretching and strengthening exercises, bracing or splinting, forearm strapping distal to the epicondyle, ergonomic adjustments to work areas, and pain management using therapeutic hot and cold. In some cases, when occupational therapists are properly trained in ultrasound or iontophoresis, these physical agent modalities may be used.

The evidence-based literature review question asked, "What occupational therapy interventions are effective in the rehabilitation of individuals with work-related elbow injuries and illnesses?" The studies examined in the review include five that examined multiple physical-based interventions, three that focused on the effectiveness of splinting, one that focused on deep

transverse friction massage, one that examined the efficacy of strengthening, and one that evaluated low-level laser therapy.

This review of the evidence provides limited support for the efficacy of physical-based interventions for the conservative treatment of lateral epicondylitis, including exercise therapy, manipulations and mobilizations, ultrasound, and phonophoresis. No definitive conclusions can be drawn from the evidence concerning the effectiveness of orthotic devices for lateral epicondylitis. Limited evidence exists to support stretching and concentric or eccentric strengthening for chronic lateral epicondylitis. Insufficient evidence exists to support the use of low-level laser therapy in the management of lateral elbow tendinopathy.

Although a number of good-quality studies on therapeutic interventions for the elbow, specifically for lateral epicondylitis, have demonstrated an array of effective treatment options for conservative management of this condition, the evidence included in this review does not provide unequivocal support for several commonly used occupational therapy approaches for the elbow. The following paragraphs summarize key findings.

Bisset, Paungmali, Vicenzino, and Beller (2005) conducted a Level I systematic review and meta-analysis to determine the effectiveness of physical interventions on clinically relevant outcomes for lateral epicondylitis. The authors defined *physical interventions* "as any intervention that was physical in nature—that is, not solely pharmaceutical or surgical" (p. 412). They reviewed 28 randomized controlled trials on a variety of interventions, including acupuncture, manipulation, kinesiotaping, orthotics, exercise, laser, ultrasound, ionization or electromagnetic field, and extracorporeal shock wave therapy. This review suggests a lack of evidence for the long-term benefit of physical interventions in general; in particular, there was no evidence that extracorporeal shock wave therapy was beneficial in the treatment of tennis elbow.

A Level I randomized controlled trial by Martinez-Silvestrini et al. (2005) evaluated the effectiveness of eccentric strengthening for chronic lateral epicondylitis.

Ninety-four participants were enrolled; 81 completed the study. Participants were randomly assigned to one of three treatment groups: (1) stretching and other conservative therapy, (2) stretching plus a concentric strengthening program, or (3) stretching plus an eccentric strengthening program. At 6 weeks, all groups exhibited significant improvements, including pain-free grip; visual analog scale responses; Disabilities of the Arm, Hand, and Shoulder (DASH; Hudak et al., 1996) scores; and scores on the Short Form–36 Health Status Questionnaire (SF–36; Ware, Snow, Kosinski, & Gandek, 2000) subscales of pain and physical functioning. There were no significant differences among the three groups for any of the outcome measures. Eccentric strengthening for the wrist extensors in participants with lateral epicondylitis demonstrated improvement at 6 weeks, an outcome that was not statistically different from that achieved with a conservative program with stretching or a concentric strengthening program. Eccentric strengthening was not associated with symptom exacerbation. This study has several limitations; exercise programs were not supervised, so noncompliance or poor exercise techniques may have influenced results. In addition, patients were not encouraged to exercise through pain. It is not clear whether the improvements over time for all three groups reflect the natural course of the condition or the treatment intervention. Four of the 13 participants who dropped out discontinued the study because of worsening of symptoms (one in the conservative group, two in the concentric group, and one in the eccentric group).

Trudel et al. (2004) examined the effectiveness of conservative treatments for lateral epicondylitis in a Level I systematic review of 31 randomized controlled trials and quasi-randomized controlled trials (excluding splinting and extracorporeal shock wave treatment) and included a total of 1,666 participants. This review included numerous conservative treatments, such as ultrasound, acupuncture, Rebox, wait and see, exercise, ionization, pulsed electromagnetic field, mobilization and manipulations, and laser. Results of the review indicate that acupuncture, exercise therapy, manipulations and mobilizations, ultrasound, phonophoresis, Rebox, and ionization with diclofenac all showed

positive effects in the reduction of pain and in the improvement of function for those with lateral epicondylitis. Laser therapy and pulsed electromagnetic field therapy were found to be ineffective in the management of lateral epicondylitis.

A Level I systematic review by Borkholder, Hill, and Fess (2004) sought to determine the efficacy of splinting as a treatment for lateral epicondylitis. The 11 randomized controlled trials in the review addressed outcomes for cast immobilization, elbow sleeve or support, counterforce band, forearm band, elbow brace, forearm support, and wrist immobilization. The review found some evidence that splinting for lateral epicondylitis could contribute to early positive results; however, no conclusive support was found for the effectiveness of splinting for lateral epicondylitis over time.

Similar to Borkholder et al.'s study, a Level I systematic review by Struijs et al. (2002) evaluated five randomized controlled trials to assess the effectiveness of orthotic devices (brace, splint, cast, band, or strap) for the treatment of tennis elbow. The authors indicated that the limited number of trials and the heterogeneity among them made it difficult to draw clear conclusions about the effectiveness of orthotic devices. The authors found only one difference between interventions in their review: One study supported corticosteroid injections over an elbow band with respect to a global measure of improvement. Injection appeared to be more effective in the short term. However, comparisons with physiotherapy, anti-inflammatory cream, or cast immobilization showed no differences. No definitive conclusions could be drawn concerning the effectiveness of orthotic devices for lateral epicondylitis.

In a similar study, Derebery, Devenport, Giang, and Fogarty (2005) conducted a Level II retrospective cohort study evaluating the effects of splinting on outcomes for 4,614 injured workers receiving primary care for lateral or medial epicondylitis. Outcomes were defined as physician-prescribed rates of duty restrictions and lost time, treatment duration, specialist referrals, and medical and physical therapy visits and charges. *Splints* were defined as "any restraint to the elbow, forearm, or wrist areas—including braces, splints, straps, and wrap bandages" (p. 1082). The results indicated that patients with splints had higher rates of limited duty, more medical visits and charges, higher total charges, and longer treatment durations than patients without splints. These differences were consistent for patients who did and did not receive physical therapy. The retrospective design restricts certainty about the causal relationship between splinting and outcomes. The differences among the types of splints were not addressed, nor were the wearing schedule, length of time worn, or extent of restricted motion imposed by the splint.

A Level I systematic review of randomized controlled trials and nonrandomized controlled trials by Brosseau et al. (2002) assessed the efficacy of deep transverse friction massage for managing tendonitis pain; the review included only one trial with 40 participants diagnosed with extensor carpi radialis tendonitis (i.e., lateral epicondylitis). No conclusions could be drawn concerning the use or nonuse of deep transverse friction massage for the treatment of lateral epicondylitis; the study reviewed showed no statistical difference between deep transverse friction massage and other physiotherapy modalities in promoting pain relief, grip strength, and functional status after 9 weeks.

Smidt et al. (2003) evaluated the effectiveness of physiotherapy for lateral epicondylitis in a Level 1 systematic review of 23 randomized controlled trials that evaluated the effects of laser therapy, ultrasound, electrotherapy, exercises, and mobilization techniques. Two studies compared ultrasound to placebo ultrasound and showed statistically significant and clinically relevant differences in favor of ultrasound, although the evidence was weak. The review revealed insufficient evidence to demonstrate either benefit or lack of effect of laser therapy, electrotherapy, exercises, and mobilization techniques for lateral epicondylitis.

A Level I systematic review by Stasinopoulos and Johnson (2005) evaluated the effectiveness of low-level laser therapy for lateral elbow tendinopathy and included nine randomized controlled trials. The review found poor results for the effectiveness of low-level laser therapy in treating lateral elbow tendinopathy. The authors reported limitations of the appraised studies, including failure to provide long-term follow-up,

blinding, or power calculations and the lack of standardized outcome measures.

Question 3. Interventions to the Forearm, Wrist, and Hand

According to the Centers for Disease Control and Prevention (2001), hand injuries are consistently ranked as the second most common workplace injury, with 1,080,000 emergency room visits by hand-injured workers in 1998. The U.S. Department of Labor has recognized hand injuries as the most preventable workplace injury (Garner, 2005). The BLS (2008) reported that in 2007 workers diagnosed with carpal tunnel syndrome required the second highest median days away from work at 28 days. Carpal tunnel syndrome was second only to fractures, which required 30 median days away from work. Injuries and conditions of the hand include traumatic injuries, such as lacerations, burns, fractures, crushing injuries, and amputations, or cumulative trauma disorders, such as tenosynovitis, carpal tunnel syndrome, and osteoarthritis.

Occupational therapy practitioners in hand and outpatient rehabilitation facilities work with a significant portion of these individuals as they enter the rehabilitation phase of their recovery. Practitioners use a wide range of treatment techniques and methods to promote healing and expedite injured workers' return to function. Such methods include therapeutic exercises and activities, splinting, physical agent modalities, wound and scar care, and massage. In addition, practitioners offer the client psychosocial support and provide adaptations and modifications to enable return to function, including work and activities of daily living (ADLs), in advance of full healing.

The evidence-based literature review question asked was, "What occupational therapy interventions are effective in the rehabilitation of individuals with work-related injuries or illness of the forearm, wrist, and hand?" The studies examined in the review include one that reviewed the effectiveness of silicone gel sheets, two that examined massage (scar massage and deep friction), five that assessed splinting, four that reviewed techniques for increasing range of motion, one that investigated the efficacy of low-level laser therapy, one that explored the effectiveness of cryotherapy, two that examined hand exercises, one that addressed the effects of pressure garments, three that investigated the benefits of ultrasound, one that evaluated cognitive interventions for decreasing pain, one that investigated workplace-based interventions, one that investigated biopsychosocial rehabilitation, one that examined occupational therapy interventions, one that addressed ADL simulations, and one that evaluated conservative interventions.

This review of the literature found evidence that several popular preparatory techniques can be effective in improving client factors (physiological and structural), leading to improved overall function (Brosseau, MacLeay, Robinson, Tugwell, & Wells, 2003; Michlovitz, Harris, & Watkins, 2004). Interventions shown to have benefits and positive outcomes include splinting for osteoarthritis and carpal tunnel syndrome and scar massage for prevention of hypertrophic scarring and promotion of extensibility of established scar tissue. In addition, this literature review supported the use of the thermal modality of heat and early mobilization following fractures and acute trauma. Other interventions shown to be effective with this population include at least one cognitive pain control technique that can be easily incorporated into occupational therapy treatment, the use of work gloves by hand burn victims, and exercise for hand strengthening and improved ROM and general conditioning.

Evidence was found that supported the use of occupation-based assessment tools and ADL simulation activities for hand therapy clients, of note because functional changes in performance are ultimately the most important to occupational therapists and the clients they serve. The following paragraphs summarize the key findings.

In a systematic review of 13 trials involving 559 people, O'Brien and Pandit (2006) found that when compared to no treatment, the development of hypertrophic scarring was reduced and the elasticity of established scar was increased with the use of silicone gel sheeting.

Two studies discussed scar massage and deep friction massage. In a randomized controlled trial, Field et al. (2000) found that scar massage reduced burn scar pain and itching and decreased anxiety and depressed mood. Brosseau et al. (2002) examined deep transverse friction massage as applied to tendonitis in a Level I systematic review and found no clinically important benefit of this technique.

Five Level I articles examined splinting as a technique for reducing signs and symptoms of osteoarthritis of the thumb carp-metacarpal (CMC) joint and carpal tunnel syndrome (Egan & Brosseau, 2007; Muller et al., 2004; O'Connor, Marshall, & Massy-Westropp, 2003; Wajon & Ada, 2005; Werner, Franzblau, & Gell, 2005). In these studies, CMC splints were used to provide immobilization to the thumb basal joint, and wrist immobilization splints were used that immobilized wrists in neutral while leaving digits free. Splinting was found to be effective for both pathologies; splints designed for each diagnosis were found to be effective, regardless of variations in style. The studies did not describe definitive schedules and durations of wear.

Two Level I reviews explored the use of early mobilization (prior to 21 days postinjury) on acute injuries and hand fractures, including 459 patients in the study by Feehan and Bassett (2004) and 3,366 patients in the study by Nash, Mickan, Del Mar, and Glasziou (2004). Both reviews concluded that early mobilization can be effective in facilitating earlier return to work, decreased pain and swelling, and preserved ROM and strength. Neither study found negative effects of early mobilization.

A Level I systematic review by Michlovitz, Harris, et al. (2004) of 26 articles found evidence to support the use of splints and joint mobilization for increasing motion in stiff joints. Some support exists for the use of continuous passive motion when used in selected postsurgical cases. In a small randomized controlled trial with six participants, Richard, Miller, Finley, and Jones (1987) explored static wrapping (i.e., passive stretching of digits into flexion) versus passive ROM for increasing finger joint motion. The authors found that passive exercise was effective in increasing ROM of metacarpal phalangeal joints and that static wrapping was most effective in increasing ROM of interphalangeal joints.

Brosseau et al. (2004) published a Level I systematic review of seven randomized and prospective, concurrent controlled trials including 345 participants that investigated low-level laser therapy for pain reduction and ROM. The results were inconclusive.

A Level I systematic review by Bleakley, McDonough, and MacAuley (2004) of 22 randomized clinical trials including 1,469 participants explored the effectiveness of cryotherapy for treating acute soft tissue injuries. This review found marginal evidence that ice treatments combined with exercise can be effective in reducing pain following surgery and ankle sprain. The optimal mode or duration of ice application was not established. Michlovitz, Hun, Erasala, Hengehold, and Weingand (2004) investigated the use of continuous low-level heat wraps in a Level I randomized trial with 93 patients.. This treatment was found to be effective in improving pain and functional status in common conditions of the wrist such as carpal tunnel syndrome, osteoarthritis, and strain or sprain.

Two reviews explored the use of hand exercise and aerobic exercise for those with osteoarthritis. Results of a Level I systematic review by Wessel (2004) of hand exercise for 314 individuals with rheumatoid arthritis suggest, but not conclusively, that appropriate exercise (including ROM, strengthening, endurance, and motor control) might lead to long-term strength changes and very short-term changes in stiffness. Brosseau et al. (2003) investigated the effectiveness of different exercise intensities for people with osteoarthritis in a Level I systematic review that included one randomized controlled trial and 39 participants. The review found no difference between high- versus low-intensity aerobic exercise but did find that both types improved functional status and that low-intensity aerobic exercise performed better against a control group.

A Level III study by Weinstock-Zlotnick, Torres-Gray, and Segal (2004) addressed the effects of pressure garment work gloves with suede palms versus standard pressure garment gloves on functional hand use in three individuals with hand burns. Results indicated improved function from the use of pressure garment work gloves with suede palms and a client preference for this glove over standard pressure garment gloves for functional activities.

O'Connor et al. (2003) examined 21 randomized and quasi-randomized trials with 884 participants in a Level I systematic review. They found limited evidence that ultrasound may be an effective adjunct for the treatment of carpal tunnel syndrome; treatment parameters, as well as frequency and duration, were not specified. In a second Level I systematic review, Muller et al. (2004) found that 20 treatments of deep-pulsed 15-minute ultrasound decreased carpal tunnel syndrome symptoms, reduced sensory loss, and improved strength and median nerve conduction. This review also indicated that ultrasound administered for fewer sessions and for shorter periods of time at each session was not effective. A third Level I systematic review by van der Windt et al. (1999) of 38 clinical trials examined the use of ultrasound for the treatment of musculoskeletal disorders and found little evidence to support its use.

In a Level I randomized controlled study, Haythornthwaite, Lawrence, and Fauerbach (2001) investigated two brief cognitive interventions for decreasing pain during dressing changes for 42 participants with burns. Findings indicate that sensory focusing—having the patient focus on the present moment—resulted in higher levels of pain relief than did distraction (listening to music), which yielded no benefit. Sensory focusing also changed the memory of the painful procedures.

Williams, Westmorland, Schmuck, and MacDermid (2004) investigated the available evidence on workplace-based interventions (described as the application of ergonomic and work duty modifications) designed to decrease pain and increase functional status in individuals with upper extremity disorders. The results of this systematic review of eight studies with 751 participants indicate that the evidence is insufficient to identify effective workplace rehabilitation interventions.

A Level I systematic review of two randomized controlled trials with 80 participants by Karjalainen et al. (2000) examined the effectiveness of biopsychosocial rehabilitation for repetitive strain injuries of the upper extremity. This rehabilitation program included a physician consultation plus a psychological, social, vocational, or combined intervention. The two studies included in review did not find scientific evidence for the effectiveness of this approach in treating repetitive strain injuries.

In a Level III descriptive study with 37 participants, Case-Smith (2003) found that clients who underwent hand therapy treatment for various pathologies using several commonly used occupational therapy techniques improved significantly. The improvement in functional performance resulting from these interventions was measured using the Canadian Occupational Performance Measure (Law et al., 1998), the DASH (Hudak et al., 1996), and the SF–36 (Ware et al., 2000). The Community Integration Questionnaire (Willer, Ottenbacher, & Coad, 1994) was not found to be an effective measure of hand therapy outcomes.

A Level I study of 36 patients with hand injuries by Guzelkucuk, Duman, Taskaynatan, and Dincer (2007) found that clients who engaged in a treatment program that included ADL simulation activities realized significant improvement in hand function, including ROM, strength, and functional skills, compared with a control group.

In a Level I systematic review of 15 randomized controlled trials, Verhagen et al. (2006) sought to determine the efficacy of conservative interventions such as exercise, massage, ergonomics, splinting, multidisciplinary treatment, group and individual therapy, and manual therapy. Results indicated limited evidence to support use of ergonomic keyboards and individual exercise. The benefit of general ergonomic modifications to the workplace was not demonstrated in this study.

Question 4. Interventions to the Shoulder

The BLS (2008) reported that in 2007, work-related injuries involving the shoulder required workers to take a median of 18 days to recuperate for all private industries, which represents the highest days away from work for any part of the body. Half of the injuries to the shoulder were the result of overexertion. The BLS reported 75,580 cases of injuries to the shoulder required days away from work in 2007. This number represents 6.5% of the total number of nonfatal occupational injuries and illnesses involving days away from work reported in 2007.

Shoulder-related diagnoses include shoulder pain, frozen shoulder (also termed *adhesive capsulitis*), rotator cuff tears, shoulder instability, anterior dislocation, proximal humerus fractures, subacromial impingement syndromes, and thoracic outlet syndrome.

Patients with chronic, acute, and postoperative shoulder diagnoses are commonly referred to occupational therapists working in inpatient, outpatient, home health, and industrial practice areas. Occupational therapists use intervention strategies to treat conditions of the shoulder complex ranging from preparatory activities, such as modalities and ROM, to occupation-based interventions focusing on client-centered roles and goals. Interventions are implemented both to prevent injury and in response to acute, chronic, and postoperative symptomatology.

The evidence-based literature review question asked, "What occupational therapy interventions are effective in the rehabilitation of individuals with work-related shoulder injuries or illnesses?" The studies examined in the review include one that reviewed the effectiveness of low-level laser therapy, six that examined a variety of therapeutic exercise interventions, sixteen that studied various combination approaches, one that evaluated a posture modification approach, one that evaluated workplace interventions, and one that examined the efficacy of joint mobilizations.

This review of the literature supports the notion that several popular preparatory techniques can be effective in improving client factors (physiological and structural), leading to improved overall function. Low-level laser therapy and therapeutic exercise for the treatment of shoulder pain were found to positively influence shoulder ROM and palpation sensitivity. Less aggressive therapeutic techniques, such as pendulum exercises, active exercises within the painless range, and tolerable functional activities, were shown to be more effective for patients with idiopathic frozen shoulder than were techniques that surpass the pain threshold. There is little evidence to support or refute conservative or surgical management of rotator cuff tears. Graded exercise therapy was shown to have a minimally greater benefit than usual care for patients with chronic shoulder pain.

Although weak, the evidence alludes to the efficacy of a conservative program for shoulder instability that includes a 3- to 4-week immobilization period followed by 12 weeks of ROM and stability exercises. Neither ROM nor stability exercises used in isolation were supported by this review. Electromyography biofeedback was weakly recommended as an adjunctive modality. Conservative methods cannot be recommended over surgical intervention for decreasing shoulder instability recurrence. There is weak evidence to support exercise and mobilization for rotator cuff disease, laser for adhesive capsulitis, pulsed electromagnetic field for rotator cuff disease, ultrasound and pulsed electromagnetic field for calcific tendonitis, and supervised exercise for mixed shoulder disorders and rotator cuff disease. Weak evidence was also found against the use of laser for rotator cuff disease, the use of ultrasound for additional benefit above exercise alone, physical therapy over corticosteroid injections in rotator cuff disease, and physical therapy alone for adhesive capsulitis.

There is limited evidence to support exercise and joint mobilization for patients with subacromial impingement syndrome. The evidence supports the effectiveness of conservative management in treating thoracic outlet syndrome that includes gradual stretching and home exercise program instruction. There is limited evidence that daily, light resistance training guided by a therapist can decrease head and neck symptoms and increase shoulder extension strength for patients who perform physically light work. There is limited evidence to support the efficacy of high-grade mobilization techniques as compared to low-grade mobilization for the improvement of shoulder mobility and reduction of self-reported disability in patients with Phase II adhesive capsulitis. The following paragraphs summarize the key findings.

Bingol, Altan, and Yurtkuran (2005) conducted a Level I randomized double-blind controlled trial to assess the role of low-power laser therapy in the relief of pain and the improvement of joint ROM in patients with shoulder pain. Forty participants were randomized to an active laser treatment group (low-power gallium arsenide) or a placebo laser treatment group. No significant differences were found between the groups in age, shoulder side, or pretreatment measures. Significant improvements were noted for sensitivity in the laser group and for some active and passive motions in both groups. An improvement in palpation sensitivity was noted in both groups. Comparison between the two groups showed better results in the laser group for palpation sensitivity and passive extension.

A Level II quasi-experimental design by Diercks and Stevens (2004) with a successive cohort as a control group sought to establish the effect of supervised neglect on idiopathic frozen shoulder compared with an intensive physical therapy regimen. Included in the study were 77 patients diagnosed with *idiopathic frozen shoulder*, defined as more than 50% motion restriction of the glenohumeral joint in all directions for a period of 3 months or more. At 24-month follow-up, 89% of patients in the supervised neglect group reached a constant score of 80 or higher, which combines objective and subjective reports of pain, ROM, and functional status. However, in the passive mobilization and stretching group (intensive physical therapy group), only 63% of patients reached a constant score of 80 or higher after 24 months, reporting no pain and almost complete glenohumeral motion.

Ejnisman et al. (2005) examined the efficacy and safety of common interventions for tears of the rotator cuff in adults in a Level I systematic review of eight randomized or quasi-randomized clinical trials that included 455 participants. The review found insufficient evidence to support or refute the efficacy of common interventions for rotator cuff tears.

In a Level I randomized clinical trial, Geraets et al. (2005) assessed whether graded exercise therapy was more effective than usual care after 12 weeks of treatment in restoring the ability to perform daily activities irrespective of pain experience for patients with chronic shoulder complaints. Results indicated significant differences between groups for the main complaint instrument and for changes in performance of activities related to patients' main complaints. Graded exercise therapy had a significant and positive effect on catastrophizing. Participants with a painful arc during physical examination perceived graded exercise therapy as less effective in restoring ADL function as assessed by the Shoulder Disability Questionnaire (SDQ; van der Heijden, Leffers, & Bouter, 2000). Overall, the researchers reported small beneficial effects for the restoration of ADL using graded exercise therapy to treat patients with chronic shoulder pain.

In a Level I systematic review, Gibson, Growse, Korda, Wray, and MacDermid (2004) sought to determine the effectiveness of conservative management as a primary strategy in the treatment of shoulder instability and to define and identify the effectiveness of specific conservative protocols. Fourteen studies were examined in the review. Results demonstrated weak yet positive support for the treatment of shoulder instability with conservative methods. These methods included an immobilization period of 3 to 4 weeks followed by ROM and stabilization exercises over a 12-week period. The authors found one low-quality randomized controlled trial that supported electromyography biofeedback as a beneficial adjunctive method of treatment. They also found that conservative methods of treatment for patients age 30 years or younger provided consistently poorer outcomes compared with surgical management.

A Level I systematic review of 26 studies by Green, Buchbinder, and Hetrick (2003) examined the efficacy of physical therapy interventions for disorders that result in pain, stiffness, or disability of the shoulder. For patients with rotator cuff disease, exercise was found to be effective in short-term recovery and long-term function, and mobilization resulted in additional benefit. When compared with placebo, laser was found to be effective for adhesive capsulitis but not rotator cuff disease. Also, compared with placebo, ultrasound and pulsed electromagnetic field therapy were found to be beneficial for patients with calcific tendonitis. No evidence was found to support ultrasound in shoulder pain, adhesive capsulitis, or rotator cuff tendonitis, and ultrasound was not found to be beneficial compared with exercise alone. Minimal evidence exists for the

use of corticosteroids over physical therapy, and no evidence supports the isolated benefit of physical therapy for adhesive capsulitis.

Randlov et al. (1998) compared the effectiveness of two types of training for chronic neck and shoulder patients in a Level I randomized controlled trial with 52 participants. Group 1 received intensive training consisting of bicycling and stretching exercises of relevant muscle groups (neck and shoulder). The shoulder exercises were carried out with increasing resistance. Group 2 received lighter training consisting of hot packs followed by stationary bicycling and stretching of relevant muscle groups. There were significant improvements in ADL scores for both groups but no significant difference in improvement between groups. Although pain scores for the intensive group were significantly lower at 12-month follow-up, no other significant differences were found between the two groups. The overall success rate was 50% at the conclusion of treatment and 60% at 12-month follow-up.

In a Level I systematic review of 12 randomized clinical trials, Michener, Walsworth, and Burnet (2004) examined the efficacy of nonsurgical and nonpharmacological rehabilitation of subacromial impingement syndrome. The review revealed limited evidence to support exercise for strengthening of the rotator cuff and scapular musculature and stretching of the surrounding soft tissues, although joint mobilizations were found to increase the effectiveness of this exercise. In addition, laser appeared to be beneficial when used in isolation, the use of ultrasound was not supported, and acupuncture yielded equivocal results.

A Level III cross-sectional survey by Novak, Collins, and Mackinnon (1995) evaluated long-term subjective outcomes following conservative management of patients with thoracic outlet syndrome using posture modification and a specific physical therapy program. Of 42 patients with a clinical diagnosis of thoracic outlet syndrome who completed a conservative management program, 25 reported that their present symptoms were better than before treatment, 10 reported no change, and 7 had worse pain. Fifteen of 16 patients who had experienced no change with previous therapy reported improvement of neck and shoulder symptoms. In total, 38 patients had relief of neck and shoulder pain, and 27 had relief of hand and arm symptoms. Participants who were overweight or had carpal tunnel syndrome were significantly less likely to report full or almost complete pain relief.

Sjogren et al. (2005) examined the effects of a workplace intervention on headaches, neck and shoulder symptoms, and upper extremity strength for 53 office workers in a Level II cluster randomized controlled trial. Patients were allocated to two treatment groups: exercise–resistance intervention and no physical exercise intervention. For the exercise–resistance group, treatment consisted of physical exercise and light resistance training guided by a physical therapist in three group sessions at 5-week intervals. The nonintervention group received no light resistance training, nor was any guidance provided. The participants simply took part in the measurements. Physical exercise resulted in a slight yet significant decrease in headache and neck symptoms, as well as an increase in extension strength as compared to the nonintervention group. The intervention had no effects on shoulder symptoms or flexion strength.

A Level I randomized controlled trial by Vermeulen, Rozing, Obermann, le Cessie, & Vliet Vleland (2006) compared the effectiveness of high-grade versus low-grade mobilization techniques for 126 patients with adhesive capsulitis of the shoulder. Participants were randomly assigned to the high-grade mobilization techniques group or the low-grade mobilization techniques group. Both groups were treated 2 times a week for 30 minutes for a maximum of 12 weeks. At the conclusion of each treatment, participants completed passive proprioceptive neuromuscular facilitation patterns and active pendulum exercises. Both groups improved significantly over 12 months. The high-grade techniques group experienced significant improvements in passive abduction and active–passive external rotation and overall shoulder function as measured by the Shoulder Rating Questionnaire (SRQ; L'Insalata, Warren, Altchek, & Peterson, 1997) and the SDQ (van der Heijden et al., 2000) over a 12-month period compared with the low-grade techniques group.

Implications of the Evidence-Based Literature Review

The following sections summarize the implications of this review for occupational therapy practice. All studies included in the review, as well as those not specifically described in the evidence-based literature review section of this practice guideline, are summarized, critically appraised, and cited in full in the evidence tables in Appendixes B–E. The evidence tables also include implications for occupational therapy practice. Readers are encouraged to read the full articles for more details. In addition, recommendations for occupational therapy practice regarding specific interventions for clients with work-related injuries and illnesses can be found in Tables 5–8. The recommendations are based upon the strength of the evidence for a given topic in combination with the expert opinion of review authors and the content experts reviewing this guideline. The strength of the evidence is determined by the number of articles included in a given topic, the study design, and limitations of those articles. Recommendation criteria are based on standard language developed by the U.S. Preventive Services Task force of the Agency for Health Care Research and Quality (AHRQ). More information regarding these criteria can be found at http://www.ahrq.gov/clinic/uspstf/standard.htm.

Low Back

The current literature on low back injury indicates that occupational therapy practitioners should be prepared to provide interventions that are direct and consultative to successfully address the multifactorial nature of work-related low back injuries. Studies describing interventions directed at the low back examined the effects of therapeutic exercises, the efficacy of client education, the importance of activity and functional restoration, the effects of physical agent modalities, the impact of cognitive–behavioral therapy, and multidisciplinary and biopsychosocial approaches.

A systematic review of the literature reveals that the evidence is insufficient to support or refute the

Table 5. Recommendations for Occupational Therapy Interventions for Clinical Conditions of the Low Back

Low Back Clinical Condition	Recommendation Level		
	Recommended	No Recommendation	Recommended Against
General low back	• Work conditioning or hardening combined with cognitive–behavioral approaches (B) • Exercise instruction combined with proper body mechanics training (back schools) in an occupational setting (B) • Environmental modifications (work site visit, ergonomic modifications) (B) • Heat wrap therapy for acute or subacute pain (B)	• General back and abdominal strengthening (C) • Participation in nonspecific physical activities (e.g., walking at least 3 hours per week) (C) • Back-school training (C) • Application of cold (I) • Transcutaneous electrical nerve stimulation (I)	• Bed rest (D)

A—Strongly recommends that occupational therapy practitioners routinely provide intervention to eligible clients. The literature review found good evidence that the intervention improves important outcomes and concludes that benefits substantially outweigh harm.

B—Recommends that occupational therapy practitioners routinely provide the intervention to eligible clients. The literature review found at least fair evidence that the intervention improves important outcomes and concludes that benefits outweigh harm.

C—Makes no recommendation for or against routine provision of the intervention by occupational therapy practitioners. The literature review found at least fair evidence that the intervention can improve outcomes but concludes that the balance of the benefits and harm is too close to justify a general recommendation.

D—Recommends that occupational therapy practitioners do not provide the intervention to clients. The literature review found at least fair evidence that the intervention is ineffective or that harm outweighs benefits.

I—Evidence is insufficient to recommend for or against routinely providing the intervention. Evidence that the intervention is effective is lacking, of poor quality, or conflicting, and the balance of benefits and harm cannot be determined.

Note. Recommendation criteria are based on *Standard Recommendation Language* by the Agency for Healthcare Research and Quality (n.d.). Recommendations in this table are based on the findings of the evidence-based literature review in combination with content experts' opinions.

Table 6. Recommendations for Occupational Therapy Interventions for Clinical Conditions of the Elbow

Elbow Clinical Condition	Recommendation Level		
	Recommended	No Recommendation	Recommended Against
Epicondylitis		• Exercise (C) • Ultrasound (I) • Splinting (I) • Ionization (C) • Deep transverse friction massage (C) • Low-level laser therapy (C)	

A—Strongly recommends that occupational therapy practitioners routinely provide intervention to eligible clients. The literature review found good evidence that the intervention improves important outcomes and concludes that benefits substantially outweigh harm.

B—Recommends that occupational therapy practitioners routinely provide the intervention to eligible clients. The literature review found at least fair evidence that the intervention improves important outcomes and concludes that benefits outweigh harm.

C—Makes no recommendation for or against routine provision of the intervention by occupational therapy practitioners. The literature review found at least fair evidence that the intervention can improve outcomes but concludes that the balance of the benefits and harm is too close to justify a general recommendation.

D—Recommends that occupational therapy practitioners do not provide the intervention to clients. The literature review found at least fair evidence that the intervention is ineffective or that harm outweighs benefits.

I—Evidence is insufficient to recommend for or against routinely providing the intervention. Evidence that the intervention is effective is lacking, of poor quality, or conflicting, and the balance of benefits and harm cannot be determined.

Note. Recommendation criteria are based on *Standard Recommendation Language* by the Agency for Healthcare Research and Quality (n.d.). Recommendations in this table are based on the findings of the evidence-based literature review in combination with content experts' opinions.

Table 7. Recommendations for Occupational Therapy Interventions for Clinical Conditions of the Hand, Wrist, and Forearm

Hand, Wrist, or Forearm Clinical Condition	Recommendation Level		
	Recommended	No Recommendation	Recommended Against
Carpal tunnel syndrome, repetitive strain	▪ Splinting (B) ▪ Pulsed ultrasound (B) ▪ Nerve gliding (B)	▪ Yoga (I) ▪ Ergonomic keyboard (I) ▪ Biopsychosocial rehabilitation intervention (inpatient or outpatient program that includes a physician consultation plus a psychological, social, or vocational intervention or a combination of these) (I)	▪ Continuous ultrasound (D) ▪ Magnet therapy (D)
Burns	▪ Passive exercise and static wrapping for secondary joint stiffness (B) ▪ Gel sheeting (B) ▪ Sensory focusing for pain relief (B) ▪ Massage (B)	▪ Distraction for pain control (includes self-selected music and music appreciation training) (I) ▪ Pressure garment work gloves (C)	
Rheumatoid arthritis, osteoarthritis	▪ General low-intensity exercise (B) ▪ Splinting for osteoarthritis (B)	▪ Hand exercise for rheumatoid arthritis (I)	
Acute injuries and hand fractures	▪ Early mobilization (B) ▪ Splinting (B) ▪ Ice plus exercise (B)		
Strain, sprain, tenosynovitis	▪ Ice plus exercise (B) ▪ Splinting (B)	▪ Deep transverse friction massage (I) ▪ Ultrasound (I)	
General hand, wrist, forearm conditions	▪ Activities that simulate ADLs (B) ▪ Individual exercise (A) ▪ Continuous low-level heat wrap therapy (B) ▪ Prevention and treatment of hypertrophic and keloid scars with silicone gel sheeting (B) ▪ Workplace rehabilitation interventions (I) ▪ Keyboards with force key displacement or alternate geometry (I) ▪ Ergonomic modifications in the workplace (I)	▪ Low-level laser therapy (I)	

A—Strongly recommends that occupational therapy practitioners routinely provide intervention to eligible clients. The literature review found good evidence that the intervention improves important outcomes and concludes that benefits substantially outweigh harm.

B—Recommends that occupational therapy practitioners routinely provide the intervention to eligible clients. The literature review found at least fair evidence that the intervention improves important outcomes and concludes that benefits outweigh harm.

C—Makes no recommendation for or against routine provision of the intervention by occupational therapy practitioners. The literature review found at least fair evidence that the intervention can improve outcomes but concludes that the balance of the benefits and harm is too close to justify a general recommendation.

D—Recommends that occupational therapy practitioners do not provide the intervention to clients. The literature review found at least fair evidence that the intervention is ineffective or that harm outweighs benefits.

I—Evidence is insufficient to recommend for or against routinely providing the intervention. Evidence that the intervention is effective is lacking, of poor quality, or conflicting, and the balance of benefits and harm cannot be determined.

Note. Recommendation criteria are based on *Standard Recommendation Language* by the Agency for Healthcare Research and Quality (n.d.). Recommendations in this table are based on the findings of the evidence-based literature review in combination with content experts' opinions.

Table 8. Recommendations for Occupational Therapy Interventions for Clinical Conditions of the Shoulder

Shoulder Clinical Condition	Recommendation Level		
	Recommended	No Recommendation	Recommended Against
Neck and shoulder pain	▪ Exercise—both high and low intensity may be effective (B) ▪ Training in Feldenkrais (B)	▪ Low-level laser therapy (C) ▪ Multidisciplinary biopsychosocial interventions (I) ▪ Ultrasound (I)	
Frozen shoulder (adhesive capsulitis)	▪ Cyriax method: deep friction massage and joint manipulation (B)	▪ Supportive therapy—less aggressive techniques (C) ▪ Low-level laser therapy (C) ▪ High-grade mobilization (C)	
Rotator cuff tears		▪ Exercise (C) ▪ Ultrasound (I) ▪ Low-level laser therapy (I) ▪ Mobilization (C) ▪ Electrotherapy (I)	
Shoulder instability		▪ Conservative program: 3–4 weeks of immobilization followed by range of motion (ROM) and stability exercises (C) ▪ ROM and stability exercises used in isolation (I) ▪ Electromyography biofeedback (C)	
Calcific tendonitis		▪ Ultrasound (C) ▪ Pulsed electromagnetic field therapy (C)	
Proximal humeral fractures		▪ Early mobilization with graded exercise (C) ▪ Self-instructed home program (C)	
Thoracic outlet syndrome		▪ Conservative therapy with graduated stretching and then strengthening (C)	
Subacromial impingement		▪ Joint mobilization with exercise (C) ▪ Low-level laser therapy in isolation (C) ▪ Ultrasound (I)	

A—Strongly recommends that occupational therapy practitioners routinely provide intervention to eligible clients. The literature review found good evidence that the intervention improves important outcomes and concludes that benefits substantially outweigh harm.

B—Recommends that occupational therapy practitioners routinely provide the intervention to eligible clients. The literature review found at least fair evidence that the intervention improves important outcomes and concludes that benefits outweigh harm.

C—Makes no recommendation for or against routine provision of the intervention by occupational therapy practitioners. The literature review found at least fair evidence that the intervention can improve outcomes but concludes that the balance of the benefits and harm is too close to justify a general recommendation.

D—Recommends that occupational therapy practitioners do not provide the intervention to clients. The literature review found at least fair evidence that the intervention is ineffective or that harm outweighs benefits.

I—Evidence is insufficient to recommend for or against routinely providing the intervention. Evidence that the intervention is effective is lacking, of poor quality, or conflicting, and the balance of benefits and harm cannot be determined.

Note. Recommendation criteria are based on *Standard Recommendation Language* by the Agency for Healthcare Research and Quality (n.d.). Recommendations in this table are based on the findings of the evidence-based literature review in combination with content experts' opinions.

effectiveness of exercise therapy and other conservative treatments for subacute and chronic low back injuries. For acute low back injuries, no significant difference was found in short-term pain relief between exercise therapy and no treatment, no difference was found in pain relief between exercise therapy and other conservative treatments, and exercise therapy did not have a significant effect on functional outcomes.

Thus, occupational therapists must consider additional factors if their interventions are to be effective and appropriate within the scope of occupational therapy practice. The research in this review strongly suggests that for interventions to be effective, occupational therapy practitioners should take a holistic, client-centered approach and should consider multiple strategies for addressing clients' needs. Interventions for individuals with low back injuries and illnesses should incorporate a biopsychosocial, client-centered approach that includes actively involving the client in the rehabilitation process at the beginning of the intervention process and addressing the client's psychosocial needs in addition to his or her physical impairments.

Recommendations based on the research support a biopsychosocial approach to work-related low back rehabilitation that includes the following occupational therapy interventions:

- Therapist-directed and supervised therapeutic exercises targeting the individual client's symptoms (stretching, ROM, flexibility, endurance, and strengthening)
- Client education (proper body mechanics, back education)
- Graded functional activity (work reconditioning, on-site interventions, graduated return to work)
- Environmental modifications (work site visit, ergonomic modifications)
- Cognitive–behavioral strategies (positive reinforcement, progressive relaxation, biofeedback)
- Physical agent modalities (superficial heat, transcutaneal electrical nerve stimulation) as preparatory or adjunctive interventions.

The case descriptions in Table 9 illustrate the application of the evidence in clinical practice.

Elbow

Although there are many methods and approaches to conservative therapeutic management of lateral epicondylitis, there is inconsistent evidence to support a method or approach. Evidence regarding splinting suggests that it may provide some benefit but that there may also be adverse effects. Ionization with diclofenac is an effective method for reducing pain, as is use of progressive strengthening and stretching programs.

Ultrasound may decrease pain for some patients, but the evidence to support the efficacy for ultrasound is weak. Deep transverse friction massage and the use of low-level laser therapy are not supported as effective treatments for lateral epicondylitis. Early initiation of ROM exercises for cubital tunnel release and medial epicondylectomy may facilitate a quicker recovery period. The case descriptions in Table 10 illustrate the application of the evidence in clinical practice.

Forearm, Wrist, and Hand

This review of the literature supports several popular preparatory techniques for improving client factors (physiological and structural) leading to improved overall function:

- Splinting for osteoarthritis and carpal tunnel syndrome
- Scar massage for prevention of hypertrophic scarring and promotion of extensibility of established scar tissue
- Thermal modality of heat
- Early mobilization of fractures and acute trauma
- Cognitive pain control techniques
- Use of work gloves by hand burn victims and exercise for hand strengthening and improved ROM and general conditioning.

Some positive effects were noted for ergonomic modifications in the workplace, particularly for keyboards, but these areas require further study. Other inverventions requiring further study include low-level laser therapy, ultrasound, and application of ice. Therapists using these modalities should be familiar with their application and desired therapeutic effects and should closely monitor client response to treatment.

The majority of the studies included in this appraisal were concerned with changes in body structures and body functions using preparatory methods of treatment and with assessments administered by the therapists in preparation for functional activities and occupations. One article supported the use of occupation-based assessment instruments, finding that they were sensitive enough to measure functional gains as

Table 9. Low Back Case Descriptions

Case Description	Occupational Therapy Functional Considerations	Occupational Therapy Interventions
Taylor, age 48, is a local delivery truck driver and sorter with chronic low back pain. He has been off work for 3 months.	■ Prolonged sitting limited to 30 min or less ■ Inability to manually load the typical 5 to 6 delivery trucks per day that is required by the job; limited to loading 1 to 2 delivery trucks per day with significant low back pain reported ■ Inability to perform previous job requiring the heavy work level (up to 100 lb of force for lifting and carrying on an occasional basis) ■ Current restriction to the light work level (up to 20 lb of force for lifting and carrying on an occasional basis) ■ Oswestry Low Back Disability Questionnaire (Fairbank et al., 1980) results indicating self-reported moderate low back disability that was consistent with test findings ■ Restriction to approximately 50% in trunk mobility for extension, rotation, and lateral flexion, with weakness in extension and rotation ■ Demonstration of good body mechanics with occupational therapist's instruction for material handling tasks ■ Physical effort testing results indicating good effort; no inconsistencies noted between self-perceived functional ability and observations during testing	■ Supervised intensive back exercise program and back-school education ■ Designed and observed behavioral-oriented graded activity focusing on resuming normal activities of daily living and instrumental activities of daily living and progressing to work reconditioning and hardening activities ■ Conducted work site visit, functional job analysis, and ergonomic evaluation with modifications made, including use of hand truck for material handling and incorporation of rest and stretch breaks during work routine ■ Incorporated cognitive–behavioral strategies into therapy sessions, including positive reinforcement ■ Applied moist heat before engaging in exercises and work reconditioning activities
Lynn, age 29, is a certified nursing assistant and home health aide with an acute lumbar strain. She is currently on light duty at work.	■ Demonstration of cooperative attitude but limited motivation ■ Slow gait with antalgia on the right ■ Decreased thoracolumbar mobility and strength in all planes of movement ■ Job requirement that patient handle and move at the heavy work level (50–60 lb of force for lifting, pushing, pulling, and carrying on an occasional basis) ■ Current restriction to the sedentary work level (up to 10 lb of force for floor-to-waist lifting on an occasional basis) and the light work level (up to 20 lb of force for waist-to-shoulder lifting, carrying, pushing, and pulling on an occasional basis) ■ Low and middle back pain score of 5/10 while sedentary and to 8/10 during functional testing ■ Minor inconsistencies noted during the evaluation for self-reported pain and disability as compared with actual performance; client was able to do more at times than she reported during the intake interview and on the Spinal Function Sort (Matheson & Matheson, 1993) ■ Score of 4 on the Ransford Pain Drawing, indicating poor psychodynamics (Ransford, Cairns, & Mooney, 1976) ■ Demonstration of variable levels of physical effort during functional testing (high effort on some tests and low effort on other tests)	■ Used an interdisciplinary approach with rehabilitation team comprising occupational therapist, physical therapist, and psychologist ■ Collaborated with psychologist and client on a cognitive–behavioral approach including progressive relaxation techniques, positive reinforcement, and biofeedback ■ Instructed client to return to meaningful activities, including a walking routine of 4 to 5 times a week for 30 min on level terrain, rather than providing a specific range of motion, flexibility, and strengthening exercises ■ Conducted work site ergonomic evaluation with significant modifications made to the work environment, including use of mechanical patient lifting devices, gait–transfer belts, and incorporation of proper body mechanics with on-the-job instruction by the occupational therapist

Table 10. Elbow Case Descriptions

Case Description	Occupational Therapy Functional Considerations	Occupational Therapy Interventions
James, age 42, is a county road maintenance worker with lateral epicondylitis.	■ Increasing difficulty shoveling "chat" (gravel) from dump truck to fill potholes due to pain in lateral elbow when he extends elbow while gripping shovel, supinating forearm against the weight of the filled shovel to move from truck bed (above shoulder level) over shoulder and to the ground ■ Pain and numbness radiating into the lateral forearm has resulted in increased difficulty engaging in his hobby of fishing ■ Difficulty with activities of daily living (ADL) and instrumental activities of daily living (IADL) tasks of self-care and household activities, including cooking and housecleaning (e.g., sweeping, mopping)	■ Fitted a forearm band to decrease discomfort during work and leisure activities ■ Provided education regarding cause and course of condition and introduced modified ADLs and leisure and work activities ■ Initiated work modifications, including changing to a lighter weight shovel, allowing for rest and stretch breaks, changing the movement pattern for shoveling from the truck, and rotating workers between tasks ■ Applied cold to lateral elbow to help decrease inflammation ■ Applied pulsed ultrasound during intervention sessions to decrease pain and discomfort over lateral epicondyle and radial head ■ Instructed in active stretching exercises to use throughout the day as needed
Malcolm, age 29, is a warehouse worker who developed triceps tendinitis secondary to frequent lifting of cartons over his head.	■ Inability to perform work tasks that involve elbow extension due to pain and swelling over the posterior aspect of the elbow ■ Difficulty riding mountain bike to work; vibration over the roadway and impact stresses resulting from unavoidable rough surfaces increase posterior elbow pain ■ Difficulty completing work, self-care, household, and leisure tasks that require him to reach overhead (e.g., washing hair in the shower, throwing a ball)	■ To avoid exacerbation of symptoms, initiated early passive movement to maintain range of motion, progressing slowly to strengthening exercise ■ Provided education in pain control techniques and therapeutic cold applied to the posterior elbow to decrease pain and edema ■ Fabricated initial splinting device for optimal positioning and rest during daily activities ■ Performed work site and job assessment to determine timing of return to light duty work using adaptive techniques and tools ■ With client, explored alternate transportation options and alternate bike routes to determine if the biking stresses could be reduced ■ Recommended modifications such as adaptive equipment and techniques to enable return to work, self-care, household, and leisure tasks
Madeline, age 54, is a hospital laundry worker with cubital syndrome.	■ Increasing difficulty completing work tasks due to pain along the medial aspect of the elbow with tenderness over the ulnar nerve, weakness in the hand, and numbness along the ulnar nerve distribution ■ Significant and unrelenting pain and numbness, especially after a busy day at work ■ Difficulty sleeping because pain interrupts sleep ■ Difficulty performing ADL and IADL tasks resulting from increasing weakness in hand, particularly in gripping objects ■ Impaired sensation of ring and small fingers	■ Applied ice pack treatments for acute pain before intervention activities ■ Provided education regarding cause and course of condition ■ Provided techniques and adaptive equipment for work to minimize elbow flexion and recommended breaks to do stretching exercises ■ Recommended techniques and adaptive equipment for modified ADLs and leisure activities ■ Provided instruction for self-management of symptoms, including indications for rest, application of ice, and resting positions ■ Instructed on alternate sleeping positions and, if tolerated, recommended wearing of a gutter splint to maintain 30° elbow flexion at night

experienced and reported by hand therapy clients. This is an important outcome to note, as it is ultimately the functional changes in performance that are important to occupational therapists and the clients they serve. The case descriptions in Table 11 illustrate the application of the evidence in clinical practice.

Shoulder

The literature review supports multiple intervention strategies that occupational therapists can use to treat conditions of the shoulder complex. The majority of intervention approaches reviewed were preparatory

Table 11. Forearm, Wrist, and Hand Case Descriptions

Case Description	Occupational Therapy Functional Considerations	Occupational Therapy Interventions
Lindsay, age 32, is an administrative assistant with carpal tunnel syndrome.	■ Increased difficulty typing on the computer, filing, and talking on the telephone for extended periods due to secondary weakness and paresthesias in hand ■ Increased stress, as she is no longer able to engage in leisure activities of knitting and cake decorating due to impaired fine motor coordination and numbness ■ Increased difficulty sleeping through the night due to shooting pains in hand ■ Overall activities of daily living (ADLs) and leisure activity performance scores on the Canadian Occupational Performance Measure (Law et al., 1998) of 6/10 with satisfaction rating of 4/10; work performance score 5/10 with satisfaction rating of 4/10	■ Designed, fabricated, and fitted a wrist orthotic; designed ergonomic modifications to work site that included hands-free headset for telephone, modified filing system, and ergonomic keyboard ■ Suggested modification to home environment, including instruction for modification of knitting technique and time spent in activity; recommended changes to components used in cake decorating to reduce static grip force and strain on finger flexor tendons ■ Provided education regarding cause and course of condition, nerve gliding exercises, carpal ligament stretch, and reintroduction of modified leisure and work activities ■ Applied pulsed ultrasound during treatment sessions before work simulation tasks to facilitate healing of median nerve
Jason, age 28, is a hydraulic press operator who experienced a crush injury to the hand.	■ Difficulty with ADL and instrumental activities of daily living (IADL) tasks, including self-care and home care activities ■ Dissatisfaction with inability to complete leisure activity of gardening ■ Inability to work as hydraulic press operator	■ Provided modifications and adaptive tools and techniques to enable return to self-care, home care, and light gardening activities within 2 weeks of injury ■ Provided wound care and scar control techniques to facilitate healing of partial thickness wound ■ Demonstrated edema control techniques (e.g., use of cold, massage) ■ Initiated early active movement ■ Taught pain control techniques, including cognitive sensory focusing and use of therapeutic cold ■ Provided splinting for optimal positioning and protection during sleep ■ Following consultation with physician and work supervisor, determined that client would return to work in a light-duty capacity using adaptive techniques and tools provided by occupational therapist
Esmeralda, age 60, is employed in a hospital housekeeping department. She has posttraumatic carpometacarpal (CMC) osteoarthritis of her right dominant thumb.	■ Significant difficulties with self-care activities requiring forceful and sustained pinching, such as dressing, washing clothes, cooking, and washing dishes (3/10); dissatisfaction with functional limitations (4/10) ■ Increasing difficulty with all work activities due to pain, weakness, and limited movement (2/10) ■ Pain, weakness, and swelling were client factors targeted as contributing to the current level of dysfunction	■ Designed and fabricated custom hand-based CMC immobilization splint to be used during activities that cause pain; client to remove splint during times of rest ■ Recommended ice pack treatments for acute pain ■ Recommended various adaptations for work duties, including joint protection techniques to decrease stress on the CMC joint ■ Provided techniques and adaptive equipment for ADLs and IADLs.

Table 11. Forearm, Wrist, and Hand Case Descriptions *(cont.)*

Case Description	Occupational Therapy Functional Considerations	Occupational Therapy Interventions
Julia, age 54 years, is the assistant manager of a liquor store with complex regional pain syndrome secondary to an ulnar nerve and tendon laceration of her right dominant hand.	■ Increased stress due to risk of losing a promotion at work that she was to receive within the month ■ Inability to complete self-care (e.g., hair care, make-up application) and household tasks (e.g., meal preparation, laundry, housecleaning) independently ■ Inability to engage in desired leisure or work activities ■ Significant unrelenting pain ■ Posttraumatic stress disorder leading to interpersonal issues with adult daughter with whom she lives ■ Significant edema creating difficulty with hand movement ■ Impaired sensation of ulnar nerve–innervated digits (ring and small fingers) ■ Limited passive and active range of motion of digits	■ Provided and fitted splint to protect healing tendon and nerve ■ Provided dressing changes and cleansing to ensure rapid and infection-free healing of surgical and trauma wound ■ Provided edema control techniques to do at home, such as use of ice, elevation, and retrograde massage ■ Used massage and applied silicone gel sheeting for scar control ■ Instructed in one-handed methods to perform ADLs and IADLs during healing phases ■ Instructed in therapeutic exercises appropriate to the stage of tendon healing and progressed exercises as restrictions were lifted (active and passive motion exercises within pain tolerance) ■ Applied physical agent modalities (fluidotherapy, ultrasound) to decrease pain and stiffness before engagement in treatment activities ■ Monitored return of nerve function ■ Demonstrated pain control techniques as needed ■ Included engagement in meaningful and relevant activities to redirect attention and enhance fluidity of movement ■ After tendon healed, introduced exercises and activities designed to strengthen forearm, wrist, and hand ■ After tendon healed, reintroduced use of the right hand for self-care, household, and work activities ■ After tendon healed, initiated work hardening program, including psychological counseling

activities, or those that prepare patients for occupational performance. It is of the utmost importance that these interventions not constitute the complete spectrum of occupational therapy interventions; occupational therapists must also use purposeful and occupation-based activities to develop a holistic treatment plan that facilitates a return to ADLs.

Preparatory activities supported by the evidence include ROM and exercise, conservative management, joint mobilization, laser, electromyography feedback, pulsed electromagnetic field, the Cyriax method, and ultrasound. ROM and exercise were supported for patients with rotator cuff tears, shoulder instability, proximal humerus fractures, subacromial impingement syndrome, trapezius mylagia, chronic neck and shoulder pain, frozen shoulder, and thoracic outlet syndrome. Joint mobilizations were supported for patients with subacromial impingement syndrome and adhesive capsulitis. Laser treatments were supported only for patients with adhesive capsulitis; they were not found to be more effective than alternative methods for treating rotator cuff tears and shoulder pain. Weak evidence was found to support both electromyography feedback for patients with shoulder instability and pulsed electromagnetic field for patients with calcific tendonitis and rotator cuff tears. The Cyriax method of deep friction massage and joint manipulations was found to be beneficial in terms of motion, pain, and treatment time for patients with adhesive capsulitis. Finally, ultrasound was weakly supported for the diagnosis of calcific tendonitis.

When comparing the benefits of surgical versus conservative management, the implementation of occupational therapy intervention was supported for patients with shoulder instability, subacromial impingement syndrome, and thoracic outlet syndrome. The case descriptions in Table 12 illustrate the application of the evidence in clinical practice.

Strengths and Limitations of the Review

This evidence-based literature review yielded many high-quality studies. Of the 87 studies included, 76 were at the highest level of evidence (Level I). Strengths of the literature review include quality control through a peer review process and the wide variety

Table 12. Shoulder Case Descriptions

Case Description	Occupational Therapy Functional Considerations	Occupational Therapy Interventions
Susan, age 37, is a businesswoman who developed subacromial impingement due to extensive traveling and need to transport heavy luggage and briefcase with laptop computer.	▪ Increasing difficulty retrieving suitcases from baggage claim due to pain in dominant shoulder during resisted abduction and extension; also reports pain in shoulder while carrying suitcases into and out of her home, which has many stairs ▪ Pain in lateral and anterior shoulder that is exacerbated by need to walk two large dogs with 16-ft flexible leashes ▪ Difficulty with ADL tasks of washing, drying, and styling hair as well as independently transporting and shelving groceries and household items	▪ Provided education regarding cause and course of condition, including comprehensive analysis of activities of daily living (ADLs) and instrumental activities of daily living and carrying positions ▪ Recommended modifications for luggage, briefcase (decreased lever arms, decreased weight of individual items), and dog leashes to ensure joint protection ▪ Provided low-level laser therapy or ultrasound to restore functional, pain-free range of motion (ROM) and decrease inflammatory process ▪ Provided exercises to strengthen the rotator cuff and scapular musculature ▪ Performed manual stretching of the surrounding soft tissues coupled with glenohumeral joint mobilization
Shirley, age 56, is a paralegal who developed adhesive capsulitis following a scaphoid fracture with lengthy cast immobilization.	▪ Inability to perform work tasks that include external rotation or abduction, including reaching to retrieve files and books in the office ▪ Difficulty, due to shoulder pain and decreased ROM, with lifting and transporting her 2-year-old granddaughter, who she previously watched 1 weekend a month ▪ Difficulty removing wet clothing from her top-load washing machine due to pain with resisted ROM. Unable to do laundry unassisted. ▪ Difficulty washing, drying, and styling hair; cannot don normal working clothes and is only wearing button-down shirts and elastic-waist pants	▪ Provided education regarding cause and course of condition, including comprehensive evaluation of pain and active and passive ROM ▪ Designed modifications of work, household, and leisure tasks to avoid painful positions and increase independence ▪ Implemented minimally aggressive therapeutic techniques below threshold of pain, including pendulum exercises, active exercises within painless range, and tolerable functional activities ▪ Incorporated the Cyriax method of rehabilitation, including deep friction massage and joint manipulation ▪ Performed high-grade mobilization techniques to the glenohumeral joint
Martha, age 63, is a kindergarten teacher with osteoporosis. She sustained a proximal humerus fracture when she slipped and fell in her classroom.	▪ Inability to complete bilateral ADL tasks, with resultant increased time and decreased independence in bathing, dressing, and household tasks due to pain and decreased ROM against gravity in affected extremity ▪ Difficulty with health management routine, including inability to drive to or participate in her yoga class; hesitancy to resume community activities due to fear of falling, pain, and persistent edema in distal arm	▪ Provided education regarding the cause and course of condition, including comprehensive evaluation of pain, edema, sensation, and active ROM of the glenohumeral and elbow joints per physician's indication of fracture healing ▪ Provided proximal humeral fracture bracing for initial 6-week period to stabilize fracture per orthopedic physician referral ▪ Initial evaluation and interventions were directed to the uninvolved elbow, wrist, and hand joints to maintain motion and decrease edema

Table 12. Shoulder Case Descriptions *(cont.)*

Case Description	Occupational Therapy Functional Considerations	Occupational Therapy Interventions
	▪ Inability to return to work due to pain and decreased ROM in affected extremity, which limit her ability to write on the board, assist children with donning coats and shoes, and carry bins of craft items; difficulty attending to tasks due to narcotic pain medication	▪ Initially provided training in one-handed completion of ADL tasks, with focus on grooming, dressing, and light work tasks (e.g., writing, cleaning) incorporating the affected upper extremity as an assist ▪ Provided self-instructed home exercise program (HEP) for distal upper extremity ROM and edema control/management ▪ Once cleared by physician, client received moist heat to affected shoulder (for approximately 20 minutes), followed by participation in early mobilization with graded exercises (with instruction for HEP), including active shoulder pendulum exercises and progressive functional activities (e.g., cleaning table tops and progressing to cleaning white boards in the classroom) ▪ Client was then taught progressive strengthening exercises that targeted the rotator cuff musculature and work simulation tasks such as writing on white board, carrying classroom items that weighed 5–15 lb 20–30 feet, and cleaning activities

of sources reviewed. Limitations of the review include its broad focus encompassing numerous interventions and variations in the outcome assessments used in clinical trials that made it difficult to compare trials. In addition, the following limitations were found in the individual reviews and studies:
- Poor methodological quality
- Inadequate reporting of results
- Selection and publication bias
- Absence of full descriptions of terms and treatment techniques
- Potential placebo effect
- Lack of ability to isolate the effects of variables
- Methodological limitations
- Potential Hawthorne effect
- Small sample sizes
- Brief periods of intervention
- Poor statistical methodology
- Geographic differences in variables
- Regional differences in treatments administered.

Evidence-based literature reviews can be considered works in progress because the research literature is an indication of what is available at a given point in time. While there is a body of evidence to inform recommendations for practice, there are several areas in which the evidence is still limited or inconclusive. As discussed in Appendix A, *evidence-based occupational therapy practice* "uses research evidence together with clinical knowledge and reasoning to make decisions about interventions that are effective for a specific client" (p. 57 in this publication; Law & Baum, 1998, p. 131). On the basis of this definition, occupational therapists use information gathered from the client and the evaluation to develop occupation-based and client-centered intervention plans. During this process, information from several sources, including the best available evidence, is used to inform and support the intervention plan and process. This approach is also useful in those clinical situations in which the evidence is limited. Maintaining careful and ongoing documentation records of the outcomes of the intervention provides important information that guides the intervention process including implementation, ongoing review, and re-evaluation. Using this combination of client-centered intervention informed by evidence, current best practice in occupational therapy interventions focuses on occupation and participation, incorporating preparatory methods as needed.

The results of the evidence-based literature review have clear implications for occupational therapy research: More well-designed studies, particularly addressing the effectiveness of occupation-based interventions, are needed. This research can be carried out either by occupational therapy practitioners and researchers working independently or in collaboration with other disciplines.

In the area of academic education, occupational therapy professional programs have a long history of guiding new occupational therapists and occupational therapy assistants to provide services to individuals with work-related injuries and illnesses. At the same time, education in evidence-based practice has become an essential component of occupational therapy academic programs. In the future, academic programs need to consider the inclusion of evidence-based practice in all curricular components relating to the area of work-related injuries and illnesses. In addition, students need to be able to distinguish between currently available evidence and areas where evidence is limited or lacking.

Conclusion

From a programmatic perspective, the literature suggests that a coordinated, case management approach to treatment of clients with work-related injuries and illnesses will achieve the best outcomes. Occupational therapy programs should incorporate a multidisciplinary approach focusing on the client's individual needs (physical, psychological, and social), performance contexts, and activity demands.

The literature review highlights a fragmented workers' compensation system in the United States that lacks a coordinated, evidence-based case management approach to dealing with work-related injuries (Schonstein et al., 2003). The literature suggests the need to develop a national data management system for work-related injury and illness that collects, analyzes, and interprets program outcomes to in-form future research, policy, and practice (Linz et al., 2002).

■ ■ ■

Appendix A. Evidence-Based Literature Review Methodology

Evidence-Based Practice

One great challenge facing health care systems, service providers, public education, and policymakers is to ensure that scarce resources are used efficiently. The growing interest in outcomes research and evidence-based health care over the past 30 years, and the more recent interest in evidence-based education, can in part be explained by these system-level challenges in the United States and internationally.

In response to the demands of the cost-oriented health care system in which occupational therapy practice is often embedded, occupational therapists and occupational therapy assistants are routinely asked to justify the value of the services they provide on the basis of the scientific evidence. The scientific literature provides an important source of legitimacy and authority for demonstrating the value of health care and education services. Thus, occupational therapists, other health care practitioners, and educators are increasingly called on to use the literature to inform their practice and to demonstrate the value of the interventions and instruction they provide to clients and students.

What Is an Evidence-Based Practice Perspective?

According to Law and Baum (1998), *evidence-based occupational therapy practice* "uses research evidence together with clinical knowledge and reasoning to make decisions about interventions that are effective for a specific client" (p. 131). An evidence-based perspective is based on the assumption that scientific evidence of the effectiveness of occupational therapy intervention can be judged to be more or less strong and valid according to a hierarchy of research designs and an assessment of the quality of the research. AOTA uses standards of evidence modeled from standards developed in evidence-based medicine. This model standardizes and ranks the value of scientific evidence for biomedical practice using the grading system in Table A1. In this system, the highest levels of evidence include systematic reviews of the literature, meta-analyses, and randomized controlled trials. In randomized controlled trials, the outcomes of an intervention are compared to the outcomes of a control group, and participation in either group is determined randomly. The evidence-based literature review presented here includes Level I randomized controlled trials; Level II studies, in which assignment to a treatment or a control group is not randomized (cohort study); and Level III studies, which do not have a control group.

This study was initiated and supported by the American Occupational Therapy Association as part of the Evidence-Based Literature Review project. In May 2005, the AOTA Representative Assembly passed a motion that, in part, directed AOTA to develop evidence-based occupational therapy treatment guidelines with an emphasis on the most prominent clinical conditions treated by occupational therapy practitioners and reimbursed by workers' compensation payers.

An advisory group determined the priority clinical conditions that would serve as the focus of the systematic review. The advisory group was composed of members from within and outside of occupational therapy. The group also provided information on the top diagnoses in each area and the corresponding codes from the *Interna-*

Table A1. Levels of Evidence for Occupational Therapy Outcomes Research

Level of Evidence	Definition
Level I	Systematic reviews, meta-analyses, randomized controlled trials
Level II	Two groups, nonrandomized studies (e.g., cohort, case control)
Level III	One group, nonrandomized (e.g., before and after, pretest and posttest)
Level IV	Descriptive studies that include analysis of outcomes (e.g., single-subject design, case series)
Level V	Case reports and expert opinion that include narrative literature reviews and consensus statements

Source. Adapted from "Evidence-based medicine: What it is and what it isn't," by D. L. Sackett, W. M. Rosenberg, J. A. Muir Gray, R. B. Haynes, & W. S. Richardson, 1996, *British Medical Journal, 312,* pp. 71–72.

tional Classification of Disease–Clinical Modification (*ICD-9-CM;* American Medical Association, 2008) in each area. As a result of this collaboration, the advisory group developed four focused questions and search terms and recruited Jeff Snodgrass, Deborah Amini, Paula Bohr, and Rebecca von der Hyde to author reviews answering each question. All review authors are occupational therapists with content expertise in the area of persons with work-related injuries (workers' compensation). In addition, they had experience in reviewing the research literature from an evidence-based perspective.

The review authors and an AOTA consultant, in conjunction with a medical librarian with experience in evidence-based reviews, searched the literature, selected research studies of relevance to occupational therapy, analyzed and critically appraised the studies, and summarized and synthesized the information with an emphasis on implications for occupational therapy practitioners. Jeff Snodgrass conducted the review of low back interventions as an Academic Partnership with AOTA, and selected students at Milligan College were involved in the systematic review as partial fulfillment of their master's degree. Except in instances noted below, they followed the same criteria and methods for the review.

Research Questions

The following four research questions guided selection of research studies for the review and interpretation of the findings:

1. What occupational therapy interventions are effective in the rehabilitation of individuals with work-related low back injuries and illnesses?
2. What occupational therapy interventions are effective in the rehabilitation of individuals with work-related elbow injuries and illnesses?
3. What occupational therapy interventions are effective in the rehabilitation of individuals with work-related injuries and illnesses of the forearm, wrist, and hand?
4. What occupational therapy interventions are effective in the rehabilitation of individuals with work-related shoulder injuries and illnesses?

For all questions, occupational therapy intervention approaches to be searched included restore, maintain, and modify.

Procedures

The group undertook a broad search to identify research reports for the review. Databases and sites searched included Medline, CINAHL, Ergonomics Abstracts, PsycInfo, OT Seeker, Pedro, TRIP, Rehab-Data, BIOSIS Preview, Science Citation Index, Social Work Abstracts, Healthstar, and NIOSHTIC–2. In addition, the search included consolidated information sources, such as the Cochrane Database of Systematic Reviews and the Campbell Collaboration. These databases are peer-reviewed summaries of journal articles and provide a system for clinicians and scientists to conduct evidence-based reviews of selected clinical

Table A2. Search Terms Used in the Evidence-Based Literature Review

Category	Key Search Terms
Diagnoses, injuries, and clinical conditions—forearm, wrist, and hand	Hand, hand injuries, wrist, wrist injuries, forearm, arthritis, degenerative joint disease, finger, finger injuries, digits, digital injuries, thumb, thumb injuries, amputations (below elbow, transradial, thumb, finger, with wrist disarticulation), focal hand dystonia, complex regional pain syndrome, reflex sympathetic dystrophy, carpal tunnel syndrome, cumulative trauma, trigger finger, DeQuervain's tenosynovitis, tenosynovitis—hand and wrist, extensor tendon rupture, flexor tendon rupture, mallet finger, radial and ulnar fractures, Colles' fracture (closed and open), multiple fractures hand (closed and open), sprain and strain of wrist and hand, dislocated finger, lacerating tendon, crushing injury (wrist, hand, and finger), burn, ulnar nerve syndrome, radial tunnel syndrome, Kienbock's disease, open wound (finger and hand)
Diagnoses, injuries, and clinical conditions—elbow	Elbow, elbow joint, tennis elbow, athletic injuries, amputation—above elbow, brachial plexus injury, wounds and injuries—elbow, cubital tunnel syndrome, arthritis, bicipital tendonitis, medial epicondylitis, lateral epicondylitis, tenosynovitis elbow, biceps tendon rupture, radial head fracture, dislocation, ulnar collateral ligament strain, sprain elbow, sprain radiohumeral joint
Diagnoses, injuries, and clinical conditions—shoulder	Shoulder, shoulder pain, shoulder joint, axilla, glenohumeral joint, scapulothoracic articulation, brachial plexus injury, athletic injuries—shoulder, wounds and injuries—shoulder, degenerative joint disease, adhesive capsulitis, rotator cuff syndrome, sprains and strains—rotator cuff, shoulder tendinitis, bicipital tendinitis, subacromial bursitis, shoulder impingement, rotator cuff tear, calcific shoulder, fracture anatomical head humerus, fracture greater tuberosity humerus—open, fracture humerus shaft—closed, dislocation—glenohumeral, shoulder strain, crushing injury—upper arm, complex regional pain syndrome, reflex sympathetic dystrophy
Diagnoses, injuries, and clinical conditions—low back	Low back pain, low back injury, low back dysfunction, lumbar pain, lumbar injury, lumbar dysfunction, lumbar spine pain, lumbar spine injury, lumbar spine dysfunction, low back musculoskeletal injuries, lumbar musculoskeletal injuries, spinal nerve root injury, spinal nerve root dysfunction, lumbar nerve root injury, lumbar nerve root dysfunction, degenerative joint disease, herniated disc, lumbar herniated nucleus pulposus without myelopathy, lumbosacral muscle strain, sciatica, lumbar radiculopathy, back pain—unspecified, lumbosacral strain/sprain, lumbar strain/sprain, L5 radiculopathy, laminectomy, lumbar spasm, lumbar intravertebral disc, myelopathy, herniated nucleus pulposus
Intervention	Treatment, rehabilitation, interventions, therapy, occupational therapy, exercise, physical agent modalities, physical therapy, sports medicine, athletic training, body mechanics, ergonomics, relaxation techniques, biofeedback, prevention, functional training, activities of daily living, adaptive equipment, work hardening, work reconditioning and conditioning, industrial rehabilitation, occupational medicine, energy conservation, social skills training, cognitive–behavioral therapy, job coaching, job modification, job retraining, occupational rehabilitation, preprosthetic and prosthetic training, edema control, limb reshaping, therapeutic management, joint protection, scapulohumeral rhythm, arthrokinematics
Outcomes	Return to work, disability, level of independence, activities of daily living, ADL, instrumental activities of daily living, IADL, absenteeism, physical mobility, functional or work capacity evaluation, quality of life, coping patterns, prosthetic use, pain, dysfunction, function, sickness, fatigue, endurance, strength, dynamometry, range of motion, ROM, electromyography, EMG, nerve conduction velocity, NCV, pinch strength, grip strength, sensation, coordination, weakness, volumetric measurement for edema, circumferential measurement for edema, depression, anxiety, psychological distress, fear, symptom magnification, occupational stress

questions and topics. In addition, the group checked reference lists from articles included in the systematic review for potential articles and hand searched the *Journal of Hand Therapy*.

The review authors, AOTA staff, and a project consultant developed search terms for review by the advisory group. Terms used in the search are listed in Table A2. In addition, a filter based on one developed by McMaster University (http://www.urmc.rochester.edu/hslt/miner/digital_library/evidence_based_resources.cfm) was used to narrow the search to research studies. The review author and the AOTA consultant reviewed the articles according to their quality (e.g., scientific rigor, lack of bias) and levels of evidence. Guidelines for reviewing quantitative studies were based on those developed by Law (2002) and colleagues to ensure that the evidence is ranked according to uniform definitions of research design elements.

Articles were included in the review if they provided evidence for an intervention approach used in the rehabilitation of work-related injuries and illnesses of the low back, elbow, forearm, wrist, hand, and shoulder; had been peer reviewed; were published after 1986; and addressed an intervention approach within the domain of occupational therapy. Only studies determined to fit Level I, Level II, and Level III criteria were included. Research studies were excluded if they were judged to be outside the domain of occupational therapy, were published before 1986, were Level IV or V evidence, used qualitative methods to the exclusion of quantitative methods, or were not peer reviewed. A total of 17,440 citations were reviewed, and 217 articles were reviewed to determine if they fit the criteria. The review authors, the AOTA consultant, and AOTA staff made the final selection of articles to be reviewed.

The review authors critically appraised the 84 studies meeting inclusion criteria using structured categories, including study level, study design, number of participants, types of interventions and outcome measures, summary of results, study limitations, and implications of the study for occupational therapy. Among the 87 studies, 76 were Level I, 3 were Level II, and 8 were Level III. The systematic review presented in this guideline synthesizes the findings for the four focused questions.

■ ■ ■

Appendix B.
Evidence Table — Low Back

Evidence Table—Low Back

Author/Year	Study Objectives	Level/Design/ Participants	Intervention and Outcome Measures	Results	Study Limitations	Implications for Occupational Therapy
Bekkering et al., 2005	To evaluate interventions included in clinical guidelines on physical therapy for participants with low back pain	I—Cluster randomized controlled trial $N = 500$ patients, 113 primary care physical therapists assigned to 1 of 2 groups	*Interventions:* Group 1 (control group) received standard passive method of dissemination. Group 2 (intervention group) received additional active training strategy consisting of two sessions with education, group discussion, role-playing, feedback, and reminders. *Outcome measures:* ■ Physical functioning (Quebec Back Pain Disability Scale) ■ Pain (Pain Numeric Rating Scale) ■ Sick leave—number of days off work in past 6 weeks ■ Cognitive and behavioral pain coping strategies (Pain Coping Inventory) ■ Beliefs about the inevitable consequences of future life with low back pain (Back Beliefs Questionnaire).	At 12-month follow-up, there was no significant difference between the control group and the intervention group in physical functioning. There was no overall difference between the two groups for any of the coping subscales.	Participating physical therapists were self-selected. They likely volunteered because they were interested in low back pain, and they may have been familiar with the latest evidence in this field. Therefore, the control group may have already read and adhered to the important recommendations of the guidelines. Generalizability may have been compromised by the possibility that mostly motivated participants completed the questionnaires. Researchers telephoned participants and asked them to provide missing data without blinding to group allocation, possibly introducing bias.	There was no significant difference between the outcomes of a standard physical rehabilitation strategy and an active implementation strategy. The active implementation strategy increased focus on an individual's ADLs to promote function rather than decrease pain. This focus is closely related to the tenets of occupational therapy. These active strategies added no additional benefit to participants' functional outcomes following therapeutic services. Therefore, this study provides no evidence that an active intervention strategy provides a more beneficial method of treatment for low back injuries.
Dattroy et al., 1997	To evaluate at-work training in proper body mechanics in populations at risk for low back injuries	I—Randomized controlled trial	*Interventions:* Intervention group received back school that taught principles of back safety, includ-	The back education program did not reduce rate of low back injury, median cost per injury, time off	Study is of good quality.	The study failed to demonstrate that instruction in proper body mechanics alone is an effective

Reference: Bekkering, G., van Tulder, M., Hendriks, E., Koopmanschap, M., Knol, D., Bouter, L., et al. (2005). Implementation of clinical guidelines on physical therapy for patients with low back pain: Randomized trial comparing patient outcomes after a standard and active implementation strategy. *Journal of Physical Therapy, 85,* 544–555.

N = about 4,000 postal workers in an industrial setting

Participants were trained in work unit groups of 10–12 that included workers and supervisors.

ing correct lifting and handling, good posture, exercises, and pain management. Additionally, therapists provided on-site ergonomic assessment and interventions. The 2-session back school (3 hr per session) was followed by reinforcement training 6 months after the first session and yearly thereafter.

Control group received the standard Postal Service training in back injury prevention, which involved viewing a film shown at new employee orientation and periodic safety talks at supervisors' discretion.

Cointervention group consisted of 75 injured workers from the control and treatment groups who were again randomized to receive training or no training after return to work.

Outcome measures:
- Lost work days
- Rates of primary low back injury
- Other musculoskeletal injuries.

Study examined the effect of the intervention program on lifting and handling

from work per injury, rate of related musculoskeletal injuries, or rate of repeated injury after return to work. Only participants' knowledge of safe behavior increased following the education training program.

primary intervention. Occupational therapy practitioners may need to focus more on environmental design and modifying or adapting the environment than on teaching individuals how to change their behaviors.

(continued)

Evidence Table—Low Back (cont.)

Author/Year	Study Objectives	Level/Design/ Participants	Intervention and Outcome Measures	Results	Study Limitations	Implications for Occupational Therapy
Daltroy et al., 1997 (cont.)			injuries to other major muscle groups (neck, abdomen, chest, hip, shoulder, trunk, and thigh) that would presumably be protected by changes in behavior as a result of the interventions.			

Reference: Daltroy, L., Iverson, M., Larson, M., Lew, R., Wright, E., Ryan, J., et al. (1997). A controlled trial of an educational program to prevent low back injuries. *New England Journal of Medicine, 337,* 322–328.

Author/Year	Study Objectives	Level/Design/ Participants	Intervention and Outcome Measures	Results	Study Limitations	Implications for Occupational Therapy
Fairbank et al., 2005	To assess the clinical effectiveness of surgical spinal fusion compared with intensive rehabilitation for participants with low back pain	I—Randomized controlled trial *N* = 349 participants age 18–55 with chronic low back pain of at least 1 year's duration who were considered candidates for spinal fusion Group 1 = 176 participants assigned to spinal stabilization surgery Group 2 = 173 participants assigned to an intensive rehabilitation program based on principles of cognitive–behavioral therapy	*Interventions:* Group 1 underwent spinal stabilization surgery. Group 2 participated in an outpatient program of exercise and education 5 days per week for 3 weeks and a 1-day follow-up session. Rehabilitation sessions were led by physical therapists and clinical psychologists and used individually tailored exercises and cognitive–behavioral therapy. *Outcome measures:* ■ *Primary:* Oswestry Back Pain Disability Index and shuttle walking test ■ *Secondary:* general health (SF–36), anxiety and depression, work status, complications from surgery (Distress and Risk Assessment Method).	No conclusive evidence emerged that supported spinal stabilization surgery over intensive rehabilitation. A significant difference reported for the mean Oswestry Disability Index scores between the surgery group and rehabilitation group in favor of the surgery. However, no significant differences between the treatment groups were observed in the other outcome measures.	Study was carried out at 15 different locations over 6 1/2 years. Some of the exercise group (28%) had subsequent surgery. Four percent of participants randomized to surgery had rehabilitation. In a multidisciplinary treatment, it is difficult to determine how the components contributed to the outcome.	Exercises as a preparatory method to facilitate engagement in occupations, combined with cognitive–behavioral therapy interventions to help clients overcome fears and unhelpful beliefs, are appropriate interventions for occupational therapists to provide to clients with low back pain as part of a holistic intervention plan.

Reference: Fairbank, J., Frost, H., Wilson-MacDonald, J., Yu, L. M., Barker, K., & Collins, R [Spine Stabilisation Group]. (2005). Randomised controlled trial to compare surgical stabilisation of the lumbar spine with an intensive rehabilitation programme for patients with chronic low back pain: The MRC spine stabilisation trial. *British Medical Journal, 330*(7502), 1233.

Filiz, Cakmak, & Ozcan, 2005	To compare two different exercise programs vs. no intervention after lumbar disc surgery	I—Randomized controlled trial *N* = 60 participants ages 20–50 who had a lumbar disc operation (single-level discectomy) for the first time	*Interventions:* Group 1 participated in an intensive exercise program in a clinic and back school (structure and function of the spine, main causes of low back pain, importance of relaxation and exercises, and appropriate postures for ADLs). Group 2 received a home exercise program and back school. Group 3 (control group) received no intervention. *Outcome measures:* ■ Lifting test (Progressive Isoinertial Lifting Evaluation) ■ Impact of low back impairment on functional activities (modified Oswestry Disability Index) ■ Presence and extent of depression (Beck Depression Inventory) ■ Pain (Low Back Pain Rating Scale) ■ Return-to-work status.	The time to return to work (for housewives, return to daily activities) after operation was significantly shorter for the intensive exercise group compared with the other groups. Time to return to work was significantly shorter for the less-intensive exercise group compared with the control group. No differences were observed among groups in the lifting test. A statistically significant difference was found in both exercise groups in lumbar flexibility compared with the control group. Pain significantly improved in the intensive exercise group compared with the other two groups. Both exercise groups had significant improvements in back and abdominal endurance compared with the control group. Both exercise groups demonstrated significant improvements in self-perceived low back disability as measured by the Oswestry Disability Index. Only the intensive exercise group showed improved results on the Beck Depression Inventory as compared with the control group.	Limitations include short-term follow-up, a relatively small number of participants, and participants with relatively good clinical conditions. Occupational therapy practitioners need to remain client centered and provide focused interventions for individuals with low back pain, as these strategies appear to be superior to more passive forms of interventions.

(continued)

Evidence Table—Low Back (cont.)

Author/Year	Study Objectives	Level/Design/ Participants	Intervention and Outcome Measures	Results	Study Limitations	Implications for Occupational Therapy

Reference: Filiz, M., Cakmak, A., & Ozcan, E. (2005). The effectiveness of exercise programmes after lumbar disc surgery: A randomized controlled study. *Clinical Rehabilitation, 19,* 4–11.

Author/Year	Study Objectives	Level/Design/ Participants	Intervention and Outcome Measures	Results	Study Limitations	Implications for Occupational Therapy
French, Cameron, Walker, Reggars, & Easterman, 2006	To assess the effects of superficial heat and cold therapy for low back pain in adults	I—Systematic review *N* = 1,117 participants (9 trials) age 18 or older with nonspecific low back pain The duration of back pain was defined as acute (<6 weeks), subacute (6–12 weeks), or chronic (>12 weeks).	*Interventions:* Trials were included in which superficial heat or cold therapy was administered to at least one group within the trial. Trials where cointerventions (e.g., exercise) were given were included only if the cointerventions were similar across comparison groups. Trials were excluded if they could not isolate the effects of heat or cold from the effects of the other therapies delivered. *Outcome measures:* ■ Pain (Visual Analog Scale) ■ Strength, flexibility, and changes in quality of life (Oswestry Pain Disability Index) ■ Disability and function (Roland–Morris Disability Questionnaire).	Two trials found that heat wrap therapy significantly reduced pain after 5 days compared with oral placebo. One trial found that a heated blanket significantly decreased acute low back pain immediately after application. One trial found that adding exercise to heat wrap reduced pain after 7 days. There is insufficient evidence to evaluate the effects of cold for low back pain and conflicting evidence regarding differences between heat and cold for low back pain.	Many of the studies included in the review were of poor methodological quality.	This study provides weak evidence that occupational therapy practitioners can consider using superficial heat modalities as an adjunctive or preparatory intervention to prepare for or facilitate engagement in occupations.

Reference: French, S., Cameron, M., Walker, B., Reggars, J., & Esterman, A. (2006). Superficial heat or cold for low back pain. *Cochrane Database of Systematic Reviews, 3,* CD004750.

Author/Year	Study Objectives	Level/Design	Intervention and Outcome Measures	Results	Implications for Occupational Therapy
Fritz, Delitto, & Erhard, 2003	To compare effectiveness and medical costs of a classification approach to rehabilitation of persons who have acute, work-related low back pain with an approach based on clinical practice guidelines	I—Randomized controlled trial N = 76 participants	*Interventions:* Group 1 (guideline-based group) received low-stress aerobic exercise and general muscle reconditioning exercises. Group 2 (classification-based group) participants were evaluated and placed into one of four treatment classifications. Both groups attended therapy for a mean of five sessions. *Outcome measures:* ▪ Functional disability resulting from low back pain (modified Oswestry Questionnaire) ▪ General health status (Medical Outcomes Survey Short Form, SF–36).	Participants receiving classification-based therapy showed greater change on the Oswestry and the SF–36 physical component after 4 weeks. After 1 year, there was a trend toward reduced Oswestry scores in the classification-based group. The final evaluated sample was small because many participants were absent because of their low back pain.	Using a client-centered approach rather than a predetermined intervention regimen is more effective in reducing disability and improving function, including return to work. Client-centered evaluations and interventions are the primary thrust of occupational therapy practice.

Reference: Fritz, J., Delitto, A., & Erhard, R. (2003). Comparison of classification-based physical therapy with therapy based on clinical practice guidelines for patients with acute low back pain. *Spine, 28,* 1363–1371.

Author/Year	Study Objectives	Level/Design	Intervention and Outcome Measures	Results	Implications for Occupational Therapy
Guerriero, Rajwani, Gray, Platnick, & Da Re, 1999	To retrospectively examine the effectiveness of physical rehabilitation for low back pain patients in a multidisciplinary setting	III—Before–after design N = 147 participants with lower back injuries mainly from motor vehicle or work-related accidents Mean age was 38.9 years. Injuries ranged from acute to chronic.	*Interventions:* All participants were included in an interdisciplinary treatment group and underwent a 4-phase physical rehabilitation program. Treatment comprised mainly supervised active progressive exercise (stretching, aerobic conditioning, strengthening) and ongoing participant education including	Measures indicated improvements in perceived disability and pain. Changes in lumbar range of motion were not considered clinically significant. Ninety percent of participants were cleared to return to work following discharge from the program. This was a retrospective study and therefore lacked a concurrent control group. One-tailed t tests and Pearson correlation coefficients were the only analytic methods used to test for change in pre- and posttreatment effects.	This study lends limited support to multidisciplinary rehabilitation programs, including occupational therapy–related interventions (e.g., back education, coping strategies, relaxation techniques, active lifestyle) in achieving positive client outcomes.

(continued)

Evidence Table—Low Back *(cont.)*

Author/Year	Study Objectives	Level/Design/ Participants	Intervention and Outcome Measures	Results	Study Limitations	Implications for Occupational Therapy
Guerriero, Rajwani, Gray, Platnick, & Da Re, 1999 *(cont.)*			proper back education, independent coping strategies, relaxation exercises, and ways to lead an active lifestyle. *Outcome measures:* ■ Strength, flexibility, and changes in quality of life (Oswestry Pain Disability Index) ■ Pain intensity (Visual Analogue Scale) ■ Leg lift strength (Jamar Back–Leg Dynamometer).			

Reference: Guerriero, R., Rajwani, M., Gray, E., Platnick, H., & Da Re, R. (1999). A retrospective study of the effectiveness of physical rehabilitation of low back pain patients in a multidisciplinary setting. *Journal of the Canadian Chiropractic Association, 43*(2), 89–104.

Author/Year	Study Objectives	Level/Design/ Participants	Intervention and Outcome Measures	Results	Study Limitations	Implications for Occupational Therapy
Guzman et al., 2001	To assess the effect of multidisciplinary biopsychosocial rehabilitation on clinically relevant outcomes in participants with chronic low back pain	I—Systematic literature review of randomized controlled trials *N* = 1,964 participants (10 trials) with disabling low back pain of >3 months	*Interventions:* Studies fulfilled the following criteria: one group of participants received multidisciplinary biopsychosocial rehabilitation, a minimum of the physical dimension and one of the other dimensions (psychological or social or occupational) was present, and one group of participants received a control treatment that did not fulfill the review's criteria for multidisciplinary rehabilitation. Interventions described as back schools were	There is strong evidence that intensive multidisciplinary biopsychosocial rehabilitation with functional restoration improved function compared with inpatient or outpatient nonmultidisciplinary rehabilitation. There is moderate evidence that intensive multidisciplinary biopsychosocial rehabilitation with functional restoration reduced pain when compared with outpatient nonmultidisciplinary rehabilitation or usual care.	The review focused on selected clinical outcomes, ignoring data on physical measurements and psychological scales. The studies examined selected participants with severe disabling low back pain treated in well-established multidisciplinary rehabilitation programs. The results might not apply to most clients seen in primary care.	Individuals with disabling back pain benefit from occupation-based interventions described by the study's authors as "functional restoration" with a biopsychosocial approach as compared with nonmultidisciplinary rehabilitation or usual care (i.e., without a functional restoration approach).

(continued)

		excluded unless they were part of a program that fulfilled the review's criteria for multidisciplinary biopsychosocial rehabilitation. *Outcome measures:* ■ Pain ■ Function ■ Employment ■ Quality of life ■ Global assessments.		There is contradictory evidence regarding vocational outcomes of intensive multidisciplinary biopsychosocial rehabilitation.

Reference: Guzman, J., Esmail, R., Karjalainen, K., Malmivaara, A., Irvin, E., & Bombardier, C. (2001). Multidisciplinary rehabilitation for low back pain: A systematic review. *British Medical Journal, 322,* 1511–1516.

Hagen, Hilde, Jamtvedt, & Winnem, 2004	To assess the effects of advice to rest in bed for participants with acute low back pain or sciatica	I—Review of randomized trials or controlled clinical trials with quasi-randomization *N* = 1,963 (11 trials) participants with low back pain without neurological deficits (acute simple low back pain), low back pain with verified neurological deficits (sciatica), or low back pain with and without verified neurological deficits (mixed low back pain). Patients with inflammatory joint diseases, infections, neoplasms, metastases, osteoporosis or fractures were excluded.	*Interventions:* Bedrest 2–3 days Bedrest 7 days Staying active Exercises and physical therapy. *Outcome measures:* ■ Pain ■ Functional status ■ Proportion of participants recovered, according to self-assessment or an external assessor (or mean time to recovery) ■ Proportion of participants returned to work (or mean length of sick leave) Also considered: participant satisfaction, overall improvement, generic functional status, well-being, and disability. Participants advised to rest in bed had a little more pain and a less functional recovery than those advised to stay active. For participants with sciatica, there is strong evidence of little or no difference in pain or functional status between bedrest and staying active. For participants with acute low back pain, there is moderate evidence of little or no difference in pain intensity or functional status between bedrest and exercises. For participants with sciatica, there is moderate evidence of little or no difference in pain intensity between bedrest and physical therapy but small improvements in functional status with physical therapy	There is no uniform definition of sciatica. Participation in occupations and activities can result in slightly better outcomes in reduced pain and increased functional recovery for clients with low back pain as compared with bedrest. For clients with sciatica, bedrest and exercise result in little or no difference in reduced pain or recovery, meaning that clients can continue with valued occupations without worry of causing harm, extending the recovery period, or increasing pain.

Evidence Table—Low Back (cont.)

Author/Year	Study Objectives	Level/Design/ Participants	Intervention and Outcome Measures	Results	Study Limitations	Implications for Occupational Therapy
Hagen, Hilde, Jamtvedt, & Winnem, 2004 (cont.)				There is moderate evidence of little or no difference in pain intensity or functional status between 2–3 days and 7 days of rest.		

Reference: Hagen, K., Hilde, G., Jamtvedt, G., & Winnem, M. (2004). Bed rest for acute low-back pain and sciatica. Cochrane Database of Systematic Reviews, 4, CD001254.

Hayden, van Tulder, Malmivaara, & Koes, 2005	To evaluate the effectiveness of exercise therapy in reducing pain and disability in adults with nonspecific acute, subacute, and chronic low back pain vs. no treatment (including placebo and sham) and other conservative treatments	I—Meta-analysis of randomized controlled trials N = 1,192 acute (<6 weeks) participants (11 trials) N = 881 subacute (6–12 weeks) participants (6 trials) N = 3,907 chronic (>12 weeks) participants (43 trials)	Interventions: Exercise therapy with no treatment or placebo treatment, other conservative therapy, or another exercise group. Outcome measures: ■ Self-reported pain intensity (Roland–Morris Disability Questionnaire, Oswestry Disability Index) ■ Return to work or absenteeism.	For participants with acute low back pain, there was no statistical difference in short-term pain relief between exercise therapy and no treatment and no difference in pain relief with exercise therapy compared with other conservative treatments. Exercise therapy did not have a significant effect on functional outcomes. For participants with subacute low back pain, evidence was insufficient to support or refute the effectiveness of exercise therapy in reducing pain intensity and improving function. For participants with chronic low back pain, two exercise groups in high quality studies and nine groups in low quality studies found that exercise was more effective than comparison treatments.	The authors rated only a few of the studies as high quality, which may have led to an overestimation of effect. The only outcome measure used in most of the studies was pain intensity (85%), limiting the ability to compare and report on other important outcomes.	Graded activity–based exercise programs may enhance quality of life by improving functional or pain outcomes. Moreover there is evidence that exercise therapy reduces pain and functional limitations in the treatment of chronic low back pain, which, in turn, could increase return to work for those with low back injuries. Therefore, actively engaging clients in exercise-related therapy for nonspecific low back pain is supported within the scope of occupational therapy as a preparatory method to return clients to meaningful occupations, including work.

Of the remaining trials, 14 (2 high quality and 12 low quality) found no significant or clinically important differences between exercise therapy and other conservative treatments.

Reference: Hayden, J., van Tulder, M., Malmivaara, A., & Koes, B. (2005). Meta-analysis: Exercise therapy for nonspecific low back pain. *Annals of Internal Medicine, 142,* 765–775.

| Heymans, van Tulder, Esmail, Bombardier, & Koes, 2004 | To determine if back schools were more effective than other treatments or no treatment for participants with nonspecific low back pain | I—Systematic review of randomized controlled trials in which one of the treatments consisted of a back school

N = 3,584 participants (19 trials) with non-specific low back pain ages 18–70 | *Interventions:*
Back school was defined as consisting of an educational and skills acquisition program including exercises given to groups of participants and supervised by a paramedical therapist or medical specialist. The back school consisted of information on the anatomy of the back, biomechanics, optimal posture, ergonomics, and back exercises. Other treatments included exercise therapy, spinal manipulation, myofascial therapy, oral or written instruction, placebo, or waiting list.

Outcome measures:
■ Return to work (return to work status, days off work)
■ Pain (Visual Analog Scale)
■ Global measure of improvement (overall improvement, proportion of participants recovered, subjective improvement of symptoms) | There was no strong evidence for any particular type of back school treatment. Moderate evidence was found that back schools have better short- and intermediate-term effects than other treatments for recurrent and chronic low back pain on pain and functional status. There was moderate evidence that back schools in an occupational setting are more effective than other treatments, placebo, or wait list status in terms of chronic low back pain, functional status, and return to work during short- and intermediate-term follow-up. | Trials included in the review were overall of low methodological quality, characterized by lack of blinding of participants, observers, and care providers; inappropriate methods of randomization; inadequate concealment of treatment allocation; and lack of avoidance of cointerventions. | Actively involving clients with low back pain in therapy with a focus on modifying behaviors to safely reengage in occupations is more effective than simply focusing on biomechanical-based therapy (e.g., exercise, manual therapy). |

(continued)

Evidence Table—Low Back (cont.)

Author/Year	Study Objectives	Level/Design/ Participants	Intervention and Outcome Measures	Results	Study Limitations	Implications for Occupational Therapy
Heymans, van Tulder, Esmail, Bombardier, & Koes, 2004 (cont.)			▪ Functional status (back-specific index such as Roland–Morris Disability Questionnaire or Oswestry Disability Index).			

Reference: Heymans, M., van Tulder, M., Esmail, R., Bombardier, C., & Koes, B. (2004). Back schools for non-specific low-back pain. *Cochrane Database of Systematic Reviews, 3,* CD000261.

Author/Year	Study Objectives	Level/Design/ Participants	Intervention and Outcome Measures	Results	Study Limitations	Implications for Occupational Therapy
Hurwitz, Morgenstern, & Chiao, 2005	To determine the effectiveness of recreational physical activity and back exercises on low back pain, related disability, and the psychological distress it causes	I—Randomized controlled trial *N* = 610 participants, median age 50 years	*Interventions:* Group 1 received chiropractic care with physical modalities. Group 2 received chiropractic care without physical modalities. Group 3 received medical care with physical therapy. Group 4 received medical care without physical therapy. Participants were enrolled in the study for 3 years, with an additional 18-month follow-up period. *Outcome measures:* ▪ Low back disability (Roland–Morris Low Back Disability Questionnaire) ▪ Pain intensity (Numerical Pain Rating Scale) ▪ Distress due to low back pain (Mental Health Index)	Results suggest that participants experienced better outcomes not from specific back exercises, but rather from a focus on non-specific physical activities to reduce pain and improve psychological health. Moderate evidence exists to support the assertion that flexion exercises are not effective in reducing acute pain, strong evidence exists that extension exercises are not effective in reducing acute pain, no evidence was found to support the notion that flexion exercises are effective in reducing chronic pain, no evidence indicated that strengthening exercises are effective in reducing acute pain, and there was strong evidence that strengthening exercises are not more	Because participants were primary care patients, they may not be representative of individuals with low back pain (such as workers' compensation clients) who are treated in clinical settings or who don't seek clinical treatment at all. In addition, researchers did not collect information on specific types of back exercises and relied instead on participants' self-reports of their exercise and physical activities.	Physical activity such as walking or swimming has a more positive impact on decreasing pain for clients with chronic low back injury than back strengthening exercises alone. Occupational therapy programs which focus on meaningful activities as a means and an end, take an effective and perhaps even advantageous approach as compared with traditional exercise or manual-based interventions.

- Metabolic energy cost of various activities (Metabolic Equivalent Task).

effective than other types of exercise. Specific back exercises may be counterproductive, and intervention should instead emphasize restoration of normal functioning.

Reference: Hurwitz, E., Morgenstern, H., & Chiao, C. (2005). Effects of recreational physical activity and back exercises on low back pain and psychological distress: Findings from the UCLA low back pain study. *American Journal of Public Health, 95,* 1817–1824.

Karjalainen et al., 2001	To determine the effectiveness of multidisciplinary rehabilitation for subacute low back pain among working age adults	I—Systematic review of randomized controlled trials *N* = 233 (2 trials) for those age 18–65 years with subacute low back pain (>4 weeks but <3 months) whose back pain was not related to acute trauma, neoplasms, or inflammatory or neurological disease	*Interventions:* Inpatient or outpatient program was required to be multidisciplinary (i.e., physician's consultation plus either a psychological, social, or vocational intervention or a combination of these). Trials consisting solely of medical treatment and physical therapy were excluded. *Outcome measures:* ■ Pain intensity ■ Global status ■ Disorder-specific functional status ■ Generic functional status or quality of life ■ Ability to work ■ Health care consumption and costs ■ Satisfaction with treatment.	Participants in the intervention groups returned to work significantly sooner than those in other groups and experienced significant improvements in subjective disability and disorder-specific functional status. No effects could be attributed to the intervention in intensity of pain. The methodological quality of the two trials was low; defects included lack of blinding of participants, therapists, and observers and failure to report cointerventions.	This study supports the philosophical underpinnings and client-centered approach of occupational therapy. A holistic or biopsychosocial approach to the rehabilitation of individuals with subacute work-related low back pain includes workplace visits and psychological, behavioral, and social interventions as part of a comprehensive rehabilitation plan. This approach leads to better results than an approach focusing solely on medical treatment and physical rehabilitation.

Reference: Karjalainen, K., Malmivaara, A., van Tulder, M., Roine, R., Jauhiainen, M., Hurri, H., et al. (2001). Multidisciplinary biopsychosocial rehabilitation for subacute low-back pain among working age adults. *Cochrane Database of Systematic Reviews, 1,* CD002193.

(continued)

Evidence Table—Low Back (cont.)

Author/Year	Study Objectives	Level/Design/ Participants	Intervention and Outcome Measures	Results	Study Limitations	Implications for Occupational Therapy
Khadilkar et al., 2005; Khadilkar, Odebiyi, Brosseau, & Wells, 2008	To determine the effectiveness of transcutaneous electrical nerve stimulation (TENS) as an isolated treatment modality in the treatment and management of chronic low back pain	I—Systematic review of randomized controlled trials Authors excluded studies in which the placebo groups received neuromuscular electrical stimulation and TENS treatment percutaneously with acupuncture and that did not have a minimum of five participants per treatment group. *N* = 175 outpatient participants (2 trials) age >18 years with chronic mechanical (persistent pain lasting >12 weeks) low back pain. Participants with sciatica or history of back surgery were not excluded. *N* = 585 participants in 4 RCTs comparing TENS with placebo for chronic low-back pain	*Interventions:* Studies compared participants who had chronic low back pain treated with TENS with control or placebo groups. *Outcome measures:* ■ Pain ■ Functional status ■ ROM ■ Use of medical services.	One study demonstrated a significant decrease in subjective pain intensity with use of TENS compared with placebo. Pain reduction was progressive over the 60-min treatment period and quickly reached a plateau once the treatment session ended. Pain reduction continued for the entire 60-min posttreatment period assessed. Longer term follow-up was not assessed. The other study found no statistically significant differences between treatment and control groups for any of the outcome measures. 2008 updated review: There is conflicting evidence as to whether TENS is of benefit for reducing back pain intensity. There was consistent evidence in two trials that TENS did not improve level of disability, and moderate evidence that work status and use of medical services did not change.	The number of suitable trials was too small to provide definitive support for the use of TENS as the only intervention for chronic low back pain and prevented subgroup analyses to examine the impact of different stimulation parameters, sites of TENS application, treatment durations, and baseline participants characteristics. 2008 updated review: Small number of eligible trials. The same outcome measures were not reported in each trial.	Physical agent modalities such as TENS are commonly used as preparatory or adjunctive methods of intervention in occupational therapy sessions for treatment of pain. Although the findings regarding the benefits of TENS for the treatment of chronic low back pain are mixed, the incorporation of TENS as an adjunctive intervention could help facilitate reengagement in occupations to support participation.

Reference: Khadilkar, A., Milne, S., Brosseau, L., Robinson, V., Saginur, M., Shea, B., et al. (2005). Transcutaneous nerve stimulation (TENS) for chronic low back pain. *Cochrane Database of Systematic Reviews, 2,* CD003008.
Khadilkar, A., Odebiyi, D. O., Brosseau, L., & Wells, G. A. (2008). Transcutaneous electrical nerve stimulation (TENS) versus placebo for chronic low-back pain. *Cochrane Database of Systematic Reviews, 4,* CD003008.

| Koumantakis, Watson, & Oldham, 2005 | To examine the usefulness of the addition of specific stabilization exercises to a general back and abdominal muscle exercise approach for participants with subacute or chronic nonspecific back pain | I—Randomized controlled trial

$N = 55$ participants | *Interventions:*
Group 1 (general exercise group) focused on flexor and extensor muscle groups.

Group 2 (stabilizing exercise group) focused on local stabilizing muscles and on contracting and holding certain positions.

Outcome measures:
- Disability (Short-Form McGill Pain Questionnaire, Roland–Morris Disability Questionnaire [RMDQ])
- Fear of movement and injury or reinjury (Tampa Scale of Kinesiophobia)
- Self-confidence in performing functional and social activities despite presence of pain (Pain Self-Efficacy)
- Self-perception of whether participant can effectively control low back pain or whether control lies externally (Pain Locus of Control). | Both groups experienced improvement following intervention. However, RMDQ scores of the general exercise group acquired immediately posttreatment were significantly lower than for the other group. For all other outcome measures, no between-group differences could be detected either immediately postexercise or 3 months later. | Sample size was small. | General trunk exercises that focus on flexor and extensor muscle groups should be considered as a preparatory intervention for individuals with subacute or chronic nonspecific back pain when designing a client-centered intervention plan. |

Reference: Koumantakis, G., Watson, P., & Oldham, J. (2005). Trunk muscle stabilization training plus general exercise versus general exercise only: Randomized controlled trial of patients with recurrent low back pain. *Physical Therapy, 85,* 209–223.

(continued)

Evidence Table—Low Back (cont.)

Author/Year	Study Objectives	Level/Design/ Participants	Intervention and Outcome Measures	Results	Study Limitations	Implications for Occupational Therapy
Linz et al., 2002	To evaluate several outcomes related to acute care work injury rehabilitation programs located within occupational medicine centers with on-site therapy services	III—Cross-sectional design N = 699 participants with multiple various musculoskeletal disorders, including cervical, thoracic, and lumbar strain	*Interventions:* No standard clinical protocols were used. However, based on what was apparently a consensus among the physical therapists, six typical physical therapy intervention methods emerged: (1) palliative treatments or methods as appropriate for pain reduction, edema reduction, or both; (2) ROM and stretching exercises in the direction of limitation; (3) progressive strengthening exercises as appropriate; (4) exercises to address postural deviations or muscle imbalances potentially contributing to symptoms; (5) education on body mechanics and positioning, both in general and specific to the client's job; and (6) a strong emphasis on an aggressive home exercise program. *Outcome measures:* ■ Mean number of visits before discharge from therapy ■ Return to work status ■ Client satisfaction at 3 months post-discharge.	The mean number of visits before discharge from therapy was 45% lower than a national benchmark (Focus on Therapeutic Outcomes database). Ninety-four percent of participants had returned to work at discharge from therapy. A follow-up telephone survey found no client complaints associated with therapy.	Authors were unable to establish from the database when individuals were released to return to work and the exact date of return to work, which would have helped determine treatment efficiency reflected in true reduction in days off work. Evaluators were not blinded to the treatment status, which may have caused bias. This study did not use pre- and posttest measures or a control group. Therefore, no inference about causality can be made.	Occupational therapy practitioners should advocate for early rehabilitation efforts to have a positive effect on controlling costs and keeping clients on the job.

Reference: Linz, D., Shepherd, C., Ford, L., Ringley, L., Klekamp, J., & Duncan, J. (2002). Effectiveness of occupational medicine center–based physical therapy. *Journal of Occupational Environmental Medicine, 44,* 48–53.

| Meyer, Fransen, Huwiler, Uebehart, & Klipstein, 2005 | To investigate the feasibility of a randomized controlled trial in a usual clinical setting and the effect of work rehabilitation on improvement to the ability to work in chronic pain patients | I—Randomized controlled trial

N = 33 patients with an inability to work due to chronic nonspecific pain of more than 3 months with musculoskeletal disorders; 21 participants reported their main pain area to be the back | *Interventions:*
Two groups: *Intervention group*—outpatient work–rehabilitation program for 8 weeks, 3.5 hours per day, 5 days per week. The goal of this group was to increase functional capacity and improve patient's self-efficacy using an operant behavioral therapy approach. The approach was interdisciplinary and included physiatrists, a psychologist, social workers, occupational therapists, and physiotherapists.

Control group—referred to as *progressive exercise therapy.* This outpatient program was administered by physicians who specialize in rheumatology. Physicians instructed participants with progressive exercise therapy (physical therapy) 3 times per week for 8 weeks.

Outcome measures:
In both groups assessments took place at 0 weeks (prerehabilitation), 8 weeks (postrehabilitation), and 32 weeks (follow-up).

Primary outcomes assessed were the ability to work in % of a full-time job as assessed by the physician, and the actual performed work status in % of a full-time job. | The improvement between the groups was not significantly different, but the ability to work significantly improved for both groups from an overall median of 0% to 50% at 8 weeks (*p* = 0.004 for the intervention group, *p* = 0.026 for the control group). | Small sample size. Both groups received rehabilitation interventions so the control group was not a good comparison to the intervention group. A selection bias was evident in this study because the authors had restrictive inclusion criteria by only selecting patients who were expected to benefit from a work rehabilitation program, and thus may have limited generalization of results. Two different evaluators tested the functional capacity of participants (pre- and post-rehabilitation), thus potentially affecting interrater reliability. | The results of this study support the value of occupational therapy as part of an interdisciplinary team for outpatient work–rehabilitation programs. |

(continued)

Evidence Table—Low Back *(cont.)*

Author/Year	Study Objectives	Level/Design/ Participants	Intervention and Outcome Measures	Results	Study Limitations	Implications for Occupational Therapy
Meyer, Fransen, Huwiler, Uebehart, & Klipstein, 2005 *(cont.)*			The secondary outcomes variables included: 1) functional capacity as measured by standardized lifting assessments, 2) Performance Assessment of Capacity Testing (PACT), 3) Numeric Pain Rating Scale, 4) Generic health questionnaire, SF–36, and 5) Spinal Function Sort.			

Meyer, K., Fransen, J., Huwiler, H., Uebelhart, D., & Klipstein, A. (2005). Feasibility and results of a randomised pilot study of a work rehabilitation programme. *Journal of Back and Musculoskeletal Rehabilitation, 18,* 67–68.

| Morley, Eccleston, & Williams, 1998 | To conduct a systematic review and meta-analysis of published randomized controlled trials of cognitive behavior therapy for chronic pain (excluding headache) in order to answer two broad questions: (1) Is cognitive behavioral therapy (including behavior therapy and biofeedback) an effective treatment for chronic pain (i.e., is it "better" than no treatment?), and (2) Is cognitive behavioral therapy more effective than alternative active treatments? | I—Systematic literature review and meta-analysis of 25 trials

N = 1,672 participants

Some 36% of participants were labeled as having chronic low back pain; 20% as having rheumatoid arthritis; 16% as having mixed, predominantly back pain; 8% as having osteoarthritis; 8% as having upper-limb pain; 4% as having fibromyalgia; and 8% as having an unspecified condition. | *Interventions:* Interventions in the 25 studies were focused on cognitive therapy with three primary types of cognitive therapy identified: (1) biofeedback and relaxation, (2) behavior therapy, (3) cognitive behavior therapy.

Outcome measures: The 25 examined trials in this study reported a total of 221 outcome measures with the majority of the outcomes as patient self-ratings (77%), including the following domains: pain experience, mood/affect, cognitive coping and appraisal, behavioral activity, biological, social role functioning, and use of health care system. | Results indicate that active psychological treatments based on the principle of cognitive behavioral therapy are effective. When compared to the waiting-list control conditions, cognitive-behavioral treatments were associated with significant effect sizes on all domains of measurement (median effect size across domains = 0.5). Comparison with alternative active treatments revealed that cognitive-behavioral treatments produced significantly greater changes for the domains of pain experience, cognitive coping and appraisal (positive coping measures), and reduced behavioral | Most of the examined trials were of low statistical power.

In several of the examined trials, patients assigned to a waiting list in one trial may continue to receive existing treatments (such as physical therapy or pharmacotherapy) that may be equivalent to the treatment control in another trial. There also was variability within the class of treatment controls, from continuing previously ineffective treatments to starting a treatment with demonstrated benefit such as arthritis education.

Long-term comparison of treatment and | The use of cognitive behavioral assessments and interventions to facilitate a client's engagement or re-engagement in occupations is well within the purview of occupational therapy practitioners. This study supports the holistic approach of occupational therapy to address a client's chronic pain related to his or her ability to perform work-related occupations. |

control groups was rendered difficult by use of waiting-list controls. Patients in these groups were commonly entered into an active treatment group or dropped out of the trial.

expression of pain. Differences for the following domains were not significant: mood/affect (depression and other, nondepression, measures), cognitive coping and appraisal (negative, e.g., catastrophization), and social role functioning.

Of the outcome measures, 11% were observations made by a researcher blind to the treatment condition, 6% were made by non-blinded researchers or therapist, and 5% were made by a spouse or family member.

Morley, S., Eccleston, C., & Williams, A. (1999). Systematic review and meta-analysis of randomized controlled trials of cognitive behavior therapy and behavior therapy for chronic pain in adults, excluding headache. *Pain, 80,* 1–13.

| Ostelo et al., 2005 | To determine if behavioral therapy is more effective than other treatments for chronic low back pain and which type of behavioral treatment is most effective | I—Systematic review of randomized trials

N = 21 trials for those with nonspecific low back pain ages 18–65

Chronic low back pain was defined as back pain that persisted for >12 weeks; trials with participants with specific low back pain caused by pathological entities (e.g., infection, neoplasm, metastasis, osteoporosis, rheumatoid arthritis, fractures) were excluded. | *Interventions:*
Behavioral treatment was compared with placebo, no treatment, or waiting list controls. Different behavioral treatments were compared. Behavioral treatments were compared with other kinds of treatment. Behavioral treatment in addition to other treatment (e.g., physiotherapy, back education, medical treatment) was compared with the other treatment alone.

Behavioral treatment included respondent (e.g., progressive relaxation, electromyography biofeedback), operant, combined respondent–cognitive, cognitive, and cognitive–behavioral therapies.

Outcome measures:
■ Overall improvement (self-reported or observed) | Combined respondent–cognitive therapy or progressive relaxation therapy alone was more effective than no treatment for short-term pain relief, but it is unknown whether this finding was also true for back-specific functional status. No significant differences were detected in comparisons among the various types of cognitive–behavioral therapies or in comparisons between behavioral treatment and exercises. Combined respondent–cognitive therapy and progressive relaxation were more effective than no treatment for short-term pain reduction, although this finding was based on a small number of studies of moderate or low quality. | The studies were of poor methodological quality; randomization, blinding of participants and outcome assessors, and tracking of cointerventions and compliance were absent in many studies. Many of the trials evaluated programs developed by the authors themselves, a possible source of bias. Statistical pooling of multiple outcome measures within the behavioral domain may have resulted in the lack of an effect in many of the comparisons. | This review provides limited evidence that respondent–cognitive therapy and progressive relaxation therapy may be effective for short-term chronic low back pain. Thus, psychosocial interventions for clients with chronic low back pain should accompany physical interventions and fit well within the scope of occupational therapy practice. |

Evidence Table—Low Back (cont.)

Author/Year	Study Objectives	Level/Design/ Participants	Intervention and Outcome Measures	Results	Study Limitations	Implications for Occupational Therapy
Ostelo et al., 2005 *(cont.)*			• Back pain–specific functional status (Roland–Morris Disability Questionnaire, Oswestry Questionnaire) • Generic functional status (Sickness Impact Profile) • Return to work • Pain intensity (self-reported, Visual Analog Scale, or Pain Numeric Rating Scale) • Any type of behavioral outcome (pain behavior, cognitive errors, perceived or observed levels of tension, anxiety, depression).			

Reference: Ostelo, R., van Tulder, M., Vlaeyen, J., Linton, S., Morley, S., & Assendelft, W. (2005). Behavioural treatment for chronic low-back pain. *Cochrane Database of Systematic Reviews, 3,* CD002014.

Author/Year	Study Objectives	Level/Design/ Participants	Intervention and Outcome Measures	Results	Study Limitations	Implications for Occupational Therapy
Schonstein, Kenny, Keating, & Koes, 2003	To compare the effectiveness of physical conditioning programs with management strategies that do not include traditional physical conditioning programs for workers with back and neck pain in reducing time lost from work and increasing functional status	I—Systematic review of randomized controlled trials *N* =18 trials for those age >16 in experiencing disability at work subsequent to back or neck pain and participating in physical conditioning programs	*Interventions:* Participants underwent work conditioning, work hardening, functional restoration, or exercise programs to improve work capability or functional status. *Outcome measures:* • Time lost from work • Return-to-work status • Time between injury and return to preinjury work status • Time on selected, appropriate, light, or modified duties	Physical conditioning programs that include a cognitive–behavioral approach reduced the number of sick days lost at 12-month follow-up by an average of 45 days compared with usual care. There was minimal evidence for or against the effectiveness of specific exercises that were not accompanied by a cognitive–behavioral approach in reducing sick days due to back pain for workers with either acute or chronic back pain.	Variations in the content and duration of interventions labeled as physical conditioning, work conditioning, work hardening, or functional restoration may limit the extent to which results could be compared. Variation in the outcome measures used may also limit the comparability of results. Differences among the participants studied, small sample sizes, overall poor methodological quality, and	Physical conditioning programs, including work conditioning, combined with a cognitive–behavioral approach, are effective in reducing the number of sick days for a client with work-related back pain. Thus, holistic, occupation-based, and cognitive–behavioral interventions should be considered for individuals with low back pain as part of an occupational intervention plan.

| | | | ■ Other reported change in work status

■ Other outcomes assessed included functional status, physiological outcomes of physical examinations, functional status in relation to job demands, and predicted work capacity, with or without follow-up results. | inadequate reporting of results limit the conclusions that can be drawn from this study. |

Reference: Schonstein, E., Kenny, D., Keating, J., & Koes, B. (2003). Work conditioning, work hardening, and functional restoration for workers with back and neck pain. *Cochrane Database of Systematic Reviews, 3,* CD001822.

| Smith, McMurray, & Disler, 2002 | To establish whether the guidelines in current use relating to intervention for acute low back pain are supported by more recently published scientifically rigorous research and whether additional consensus regarding intervention for acute low back pain has been forthcoming in the past | I—Systematic review of randomized controlled trials

N = 18 trials for those with acute low back pain | *Interventions:*
Interventions included bedrest, drug therapy, traction, spinal manipulation, exercise, back schools, work hardening, work conditioning, vocational intervention, and multidisciplinary pain programs including primarily psychological interventions.

Outcome measures:
■ Pain
■ Functional status
■ Employment status
■ Quality of life. | Bedrest was found not to be an effective intervention for low back pain. Limited evidence was found to support traditional exercise-based therapy. The evidence did not support the use of traction and exercise or establish the efficacy of back schools. Work conditioning seems promising, but results are inconclusive. | Multidisciplinary programs that include a psychological component show a promising trend. Thus, reengaging in occupations (rather than bedrest) and addressing psychological sequelae (rather than solely physical impairments) of acute low back pain, which are within the scope of occupational therapy practice, have limited support. |

Reference: Smith, D., McMurray, N., & Disler, P. (2002). Early intervention for acute back injury: Can we finally develop an evidence-based approach? *Clinical Rehabilitation, 16,* 1–11.

(continued)

Evidence Table—Low Back (cont.)

Author/Year	Study Objectives	Level/Design/ Participants	Intervention and Outcome Measures	Results	Study Limitations	Implications for Occupational Therapy
Staal et al., 2004	To determine the effectiveness of a behavior-oriented graded activity program compared with usual care	I—Single-blind randomized controlled trial *N* = 134 participants absent from work because of low back pain randomly assigned to either graded activity or usual care	*Interventions:* Group 1 received 1 session 2 times per week of graded activity, including physical exercise, application of operant conditioning, behavioral principles, and improved functioning and safe return to work even if pain persists. The sessions continued until full return to work for a maximum of 3 months. Group 2 received usual care, including the usual guidance and advice from the occupational physician and treatment from various caregivers. *Outcome measures:* ▪ Days absent from work ▪ Functional status (Roland–Morris Disability Questionnaire) ▪ Physical activity at baseline (Baecke Questionnaire) ▪ Pain intensity (Pain Numeric Rating Scale).	The median number of days absent from work because of low back pain was 58 days in the graded activity group and 87 days in the usual care group, a statistically significant difference. Functional status results showed a nonsignificant tendency toward improvement with graded activity. Interventions did not have a statistically significant impact on pain severity.	This study did not control for potential confounders such as compensation, legal issues, and workplace culture, possibly affecting the results.	Simulated occupational activities that are meaningful to the client are mportant in rehabilitaton and can significantly reduce the number of days absent from work.

Reference: Staal, J., Hlobil, H., Twisk, J., Smid, T., Köke, A., & van Mechelen, W. (2004). Graded activity for low back pain in occupational health care. *Annals of Internal Medicine, 140,* 77–85.

Appendix C.
Evidence Table — Elbow

Evidence Table—Elbow

Author/Year	Study Objectives	Level/Design/ Participants	Intervention and Outcome Measures	Results	Study Limitations	Implications for Occupational Therapy
Bisset, Paungmali, Vicenzino, & Beller, 2005	To determine the effectiveness of physical interventions for lateral epicondylitis	I— Systematic review of randomized controlled trials *N* = 28 trials for those with lateral epicondylitis	*Interventions:* Physical interventions reviewed include exercise, manipulative therapy, ultrasound, and a combined physical approach. Studies comparing a physical intervention with corticosteroid injections of nonsteroidal anti-inflammatory drugs (NSAIDs) were included, but those involving surgery were not. *Outcome measures:* ▪ Pain scores (Visual Analogue Scale, ordinal point system) ▪ Grip strength (maximum grip strength, pain-free grip strength) ▪ Treatment success (global improvement or participant satisfaction scale).	Most studies included exercise as a cointervention, so the results cannot be attributed solely to exercise. The only study that specifically evaluated an exercise program suggested that exercise may improve pain from lateral epicondylitis but does not improve grip strength. Low-quality evidence was found of positive initial effects in favor of elbow manipulative therapy techniques. Five studies of ultrasound provided insufficient evidence to support or refute its use as a unimodal treatment for lateral epicondylitis. Evidence from one study indicated a marginal advantage over the long term in using a combined physical approach (deep friction massage, ultrasound, and exercise) compared with corticosteroid injection but not compared with a wait-and-see (no treatment) condition.	Only 1 reviewer identified and screened all articles for inclusion; conclusions drawn were dependent on the reviewer's views of clinical relevancy of results, quality of assessment schema used, and 50% acceptable quality level.	There is insufficient evidence to establish whether nonelectrotherapeutic interventions or electrotherapeutic interventions should be used for the treatment of lateral epicondylitis. Although ultrasound and ionization have shown some short-term benefit, none of the interventions reviewed demonstrated any long-term benefits. Because of the limited evidence and the cost of treatment, further research should focus on whether the perceived temporary relief of symptoms outweighs the cost of treatment.

No evidence was found for laser and extracorporeal shock wave therapy, and the evidence was mixed regarding orthotics, electromagnetic field therapy, and short-term benefits of ionization.

Reference: Bisset, L., Paungmali, A., Vicenzino, B., & Beller, E. (2005). A systematic review and meta-analysis of clinical trials on physical interventions for lateral epicon-dylalgia. *British Journal of Sports Medicine, 39,* 411–422.

| Borkholder, Hill, & Fess, 2004 | To confirm or refute the efficacy of splints in the treatment of lateral epicondylitis | I—Systematic review of randomized controlled trials

N = 11 trials for those with lateral epicon-dylitis | *Interventions:* Participants were treated with 12 different splints representing 8 separate location-direction and purpose categories.

Outcome measures:
■ Strength
■ Reduction of load on epicondyle
■ Pain. | One trial documented the positive effects of immobilization and rest in treating participants with an elbow-flexion, forearm-neutral, wrist-neutral immobilization splint. The immediate effects of an elastic elbow flexion restriction splint on pain were not significant.

Three trials demonstrated increases in grip or wrist strength using inelastic non-articular proximal forearm splints. There is some evidence that, although this type of splint may not provide any immediate pain relief, it may provide some relief over time. In contrast, elastic non-articular proximal forearm splints produced no significant difference in grip strength or wrist strength. | None of the included studies had follow-up times >4 weeks. Many of the studies lacked sample and power analyses. Some sample sizes were not specified. Only three studies addressed reliability and validity of outcome measurement instruments. Data could not be pooled because of inconsistency in randomization techniques, use of control groups, measurement tools, and statistical analyses. | There is some support for the use of splints in the treatment of lateral epicondylitis; however, the support is not conclusive. Future research needs to focus on more accurately defining physical characteristics of splints and outcome measures as well as on using adequate research designs and control groups. |

(continued)

Evidence Table—Elbow (cont.)

Author/Year	Study Objectives	Level/Design/ Participants	Intervention and Outcome Measures	Results	Study Limitations	Implications for Occupational Therapy
Borkholder, Hill, & Fess, 2004 (cont.)				There was no statistically significant difference in pain relief when comparing manipulation with a combination of interventions including splinting and manipulation. Nonarticular forearm splints provided statistically significant reduction in load at the lateral epicondyle compared with two other types of splint and no-splint conditions.

Evidence from one study suggests that wearing wrist immobilization splints decreases grip strength and may reduce muscle activity of the wrist extensors. | | |

Reference: Borkholder, C. D., Hill, V. A., & Fess, E. E. (2004). The efficacy of splinting for lateral epicondylitis: A systematic review. *Journal of Hand Therapy, 17,* 181–199.

| Brosseau et al., 2002 | To assess the efficacy of deep transverse friction massage in treating tendinitis | I—Systematic review of randomized controlled trials

N = 2 trials with tendinitis | *Interventions:* Outcomes of treatment with deep transverse friction massage were compared with those of other physiotherapy interventions.

Outcome measures:
■ Pain relief
■ Grip strength
■ Functional status measures. | One of the studies examined the efficacy of deep transverse friction massage as a treatment for extensor carpi radialis tendinitis and found no significant difference in pain intensity, grip strength, or functional status after nine consecutive sessions combined with other modalities. There is no evidence to sug- | There was a lack of randomized trials examining the efficacy of deep transverse friction massage to treat tendinitis using validated outcome measures and high-quality reporting methods. | There is no evidence of clinically important benefits of using deep transverse friction massage for treating tendinitis. |

Author/Year	Purpose	Study Design/Participants	Intervention/Outcome Measures	Results	Conclusions
				gest that this treatment combined with other physiotherapy modalities reduces tendinitis symptoms compared with control groups.	

Reference: Brosseau, L., Casimiro, L., Milne, S., Robinson, V. A., Shea, B. J., Tugwell, P., et al. (2002). Deep transverse friction massage for treating tendonitis. *Cochrane Database of Systematic Reviews, 4,* CD003528.

Author/Year	Purpose	Study Design/Participants	Intervention/Outcome Measures	Results	Conclusions
Derebery, Devenport, Giang, & Fogarty, 2005	To evaluate the effects of splinting on outcomes for injured workers with epicondylitis	II—Retrospective cohort study *N* = 4,614 injured workers treated with splinting for lateral or medial epicondylitis	*Intervention:* Participants were treated with splinting. *Outcome measures:* ▪ Physician-prescribed rates of duty restrictions ▪ Lost time from work ▪ Treatment duration ▪ Specialist referrals ▪ Medical and physical therapy visits and charges.	Participants who received splints had higher rates of limited duty, more medical visits and charges, higher total charges, and longer treatment durations than participants without splints. Thus, the use of splints does not necessarily lead to better outcomes and may have adverse effects in treating epicondylitis.	The retrospective design restricts certainty about the causal relationship between splinting and outcomes. Differences among the types of splints were not addressed, and wearing schedule, length of time worn, and extent of restricted motion were not described.

Reference: Derebery, V. J., Devenport, J. N., Giang, G. M., & Fogarty, W. T. (2005). The effects of splinting on outcomes for epicondylitis. *Archives of Physical Medicine and Rehabilitation, 86,* 1081–1088.

Author/Year	Purpose	Study Design/Participants	Intervention/Outcome Measures	Results	Conclusions
Martinez-Silvestrini et al., 2005	To evaluate the effectiveness of eccentric strengthening in the treatment of lateral epicondylitis	I—Randomized controlled trial *N* = 94 participants with chronic lateral epicondylitis (81 completed the study) Participants were randomly allocated to 3 groups: stretching (conservative treatment), concentric	*Interventions:* All groups engaged in a 6-week exercise program after receiving instruction on icing, stretching, and avoidance of aggravating activities. Strengthening groups received instruction on isolated concentric and eccentric wrist extensor strengthening.	At 6 weeks, all groups exhibited significant improvement in the outcomes of pain-free grip, Visual Analog Scale scores, DASH scores, and SF-36 subscales of pain and physical functioning. There were no significant differences in improvement among the 3 groups. Because clients with lateral epicondylitis improve over time, it	Stretching alone or in combination with eccentric or concentric strengthening may result in better outcomes for clients diagnosed with lateral epicondylitis. More study is needed to determine longer term effects of strengthening compared with the

(continued)

Evidence Table—Elbow *(cont.)*

Author/Year	Study Objectives	Level/Design/ Participants	Intervention and Outcome Measures	Results	Study Limitations	Implications for Occupational Therapy
Martinez-Silvestrini et al., 2005 *(cont.)*		strengthening with stretching, or eccentric strengthening with stretching.	*Outcome measures:* ■ Pain-free grip strength ■ Participant ratings of functioning (Forearm Evaluation Questionnaire; Disabilities of the Arm, Shoulder, and Hand [DASH], Short Form 36 [SF–36]; Visual Analog Scale).		is not clear whether the improvements noted are attributable to the natural course of the condition or the treatment intervention.	natural course of the condition.

Reference: Martinez-Silvestrini, J. A., Newcomer, K. L., Gay, R. E., Schaefer, M. P., Kortebein, P., & Arendt, K. W. (2005). Chronic lateral epicondylitis: Comparative effectiveness of a home exercise program including stretching alone versus stretching supplemented with eccentric or concentric strengthening. *Journal of Hand Therapy, 18*, 411–419.

Author/Year	Study Objectives	Level/Design/ Participants	Intervention and Outcome Measures	Results	Study Limitations	Implications for Occupational Therapy
Smidt et al., 2003	To evaluate the effectiveness of physiotherapy for lateral epicondylitis of the elbow	I—Systematic review of randomized controlled trials N = 23 trials with lateral epicondylitis	*Interventions:* Physiotherapy interventions included laser therapy, ultrasound treatment, electrotherapy, and exercise and mobilization techniques. *Outcome measures:* ■ Pain ■ Global improvement.	Three studies comparing ultrasound with placebo provide weak evidence for the benefits of ultrasound for treatment of lateral epicondylitis. The 7 studies that compared ultrasound with other active interventions provided insufficient evidence in favor of ultrasound over any other intervention. This review provides insufficient evidence of the effectiveness of electrotherapy, laser, and exercise and mobilization techniques in the treatment of lateral epicondylitis.	Pooling of data was not possible for most interventions because of insufficient data or clinical or statistical heterogeneity.	Ultrasound resulted in significant and clinically relevant benefits compared with placebo ultrasound. The evidence was inconclusive regarding the benefit or lack of effect of other physiotherapy treatments.

Reference: Smidt, N., Assendelft, W. J. J., Arola, H., Malmivaara, A., Green, S., Buchbinder, R., et al. (2003). Effectiveness of physiotherapy for lateral epicondylitis: A systematic review. *Annals of Medicine, 35*, 51–62.

Stasinopoulos & Johnson, 2005	To determine the effectiveness of low-level laser therapy (LLLT) in the management of lateral elbow tendinopathy	I—Systematic review of randomized controlled trials *N* = 9 trials with lateral elbow tendinopathy treated with LLLT	*Intervention:* Participants were treated with LLLT. *Outcome measures:* ▪ Pain ▪ Function.	The studies in this review had satisfactory methodology, but the results provided evidence of neither benefits nor lack of effects of LLLT for treatment of lateral elbow tendinopathy. There is little evidence to support the use of LLLT as the sole treatment for this condition.	Although the quality of the studies was satisfactory overall, methodological shortcomings limited pooling of data and drawing of conclusions.	LLLT should not be used as a sole treatment for lateral elbow tendinopathy until the optimal treatment dose can be defined.

Reference: Stasinopoulos, D. I., & Johnson, J. I. (2005). Effectiveness of low-level laser therapy for lateral elbow tendinopathy. *Photomedicine and Laser Surgery, 23,* 425–430.

Struijs et al., 2002	To assess the effectiveness of orthotic devices for the treatment of tennis elbow (lateral epicondylitis)	I—Systematic review of randomized clinical controlled trials *N* = 5 trials for those treated with orthotic devices for lateral epicondylitis	*Interventions:* Participants were treated with an orthotic device in the form of a brace, splint, cast, band, or strap. *Outcome measures:* ▪ Pain ▪ Global measure of improvement ▪ Elbow-specific functional status ▪ Maximum grip strength ▪ Pain-free grip strength ▪ Generic functional status ▪ Pressure pain on the lateral epicondyle.	Of the four studies that compared orthotic devices with other conservative treatment, none provided conclusive evidence to support the use of orthotic devices over conservative treatments. The three studies addressing the additive use of an orthotic device did not demonstrate significant differences in pain perception or grip strength. Only one study compared two types of orthotic devices and found no significant differences in the global measure of improvement or pain-free grip strength.	The heterogeneity of the studies did not permit pooling of data and made it difficult to draw conclusions. The number of studies was small, and each had had design limitations.	Orthotic devices are commonly used as treatments for lateral epicondylitis; however, the evidence does not support application of these devices to treat this diagnosis.

Reference: Struijs, P. A., Smidt, N. N., Arola, H., van Dijk, C. N., Buchbinder, R., & Assendelft, W. J. J. (2002). Orthotic devices for the treatment of tennis elbow. *Cochrane Database of Systematic Reviews, 1,* CD001821.

(continued)

Evidence Table—Elbow (cont.)

Author/Year	Study Objectives	Level/Design/ Participants	Intervention and Outcome Measures	Results	Study Limitations	Implications for Occupational Therapy
Trudel et al., 2004	To determine the effectiveness of conservative treatments for lateral epicondylitis	I—Systematic review of randomized controlled trials *N* = 1,666 (31 trials) for those with lateral epicondylitis	*Interventions:* Conservative treatments included ultrasound, exercise, ionization, pulsed electromagnetic field, mobilization and manipulations, and laser therapy. *Outcome measures:* ■ Pain ■ Function.	Four studies found that ultrasound alone or in combination with other treatments could decrease pain. In two additional studies, progressive exercise therapy was found to be more beneficial than ultrasound in acute and chronic lateral epicondylitis. One study revealed that ultrasound, friction massage, and exercise were the best option for long-term improvement, followed by a wait-and-see approach. Four studies found that progressive strengthening and stretching programs produced significantly greater reductions in pain than alternative treatments, and one study found that these programs resulted in increased grip strength. Two studies indicated that ionization with diclofenac significantly reduced pain compared with the other treatments. One study found that mobilization of the radial head and the neural tension technique	Limitations include lack of blinding procedures, lack of standardized outcome measures, and lack of clear description of the techniques used.	Limited evidence supports the conservative management of lateral epicondylitis with a variety of commonly used physicstherapy approaches, including ultrasound, exercise, ionization, electromagnetic field, and mobilization and manipulations.

Author/Year	Purpose	Design/Level	Interventions	Results	Conclusions/Comments
				were superior to standard treatments, and another demonstrated a hypoanalgesic effect of mobilization during and after treatment. One study found that manipulation alone was as effective as manipulation combined with a forearm strap and the use of anti-inflammatory cream, and another study found that corticosteroid injections were more effective than deep transverse friction massage and Mills manipulation for short-term pain relief. No evidence of significant benefit was observed for laser and pulsed electromagnetic field.	

Reference: Trudel, D., Duley, J., Zastrow, I., Kerr, E. W., Davidson, R., & MacDermid, J. C. (2004). Rehabilitation for patients with lateral epicondylitis: A systematic review. *Journal of Hand Therapy, 17,* 243–266.

Author/Year	Purpose	Design	Interventions	Results	Conclusions/Comments
Van de Streek, van der Schans, de Greef, & Postema, 2004	To compare the effect of a Thämert fore-arm–hand splint with an elbow band for the treatment of lateral epicondylitis	I—Randomized clinical trial *N* = 43 participants with tennis elbow who had symptoms for >3 weeks and no other medical conditions	*Interventions:* Participants in Group 1 wore an elbow band under the lateral epicondyle; those in Group 2 wore a Thämert orthoflex splint to keep the wrist in slight dorsiflexion. Participants were instructed to wear their orthotics as much as possible for 6 weeks.	Six participants wore their orthotics <4 weeks and reported the device did not allow them to execute their work or caused skin irritation. No significant differences were found between groups for pain score or maximal grip strength. Changes in functional limitations and symptom relapse	The Thämert brace was cumbersome, which may have affected wearing time (5 participants wore it <4 weeks, compared with 1 participant in the simple band group). Job characteristics may have influenced the results. The simple elbow band is as effective as the Thämert splint, which is more cumbersome.

(continued)

Evidence Table—Elbow (cont.)

Author/Year	Study Objectives	Level/Design/ Participants	Intervention and Outcome Measures	Results	Study Limitations	Implications for Occupational Therapy
Van de Streek, van der Schans, de Greef, & Postema, 2004 *(cont.)*			*Outcome measures:* • Maximal grip strength with pain score • Functional limitations and symptom relapse (Patient-Rated Forearm Evaluation Questionnaire).	were not significant. Thus, the Thämert splint was not more effective than the simple elbow band as a treatment for lateral epicondylitis.		

Reference: Van de Streek, M. D., van der Schans, C. P., de Greef, M. G. H., & Postema, K. (2004). The effect of a forearm/hand splint compared with an elbow band as a treatment for lateral epicondylitis. *Prosthetics and Orthotics International, 28*, 183–189.

Author/Year	Study Objectives	Level/Design/ Participants	Intervention and Outcome Measures	Results	Study Limitations	Implications for Occupational Therapy
Warwick & Seradge, 1995	To evaluate the effects of early vs. late range of motion exercises following cubital tunnel release and medial epicondylectomy	I—Randomized clinical trial *N* = 57 participants who had undergone cubital tunnel release and medial epicondylectomy Participants were consecutive cases over a 2-year period and were randomly divided into two groups. Group 1 participants were instructed to wear their slings and to move their elbows only to a comfortable point postoperatively. They started physical therapy 14 days postoperatively. Group 2 participants started active range of motion on the day of surgery and physical therapy 3 days postoperatively.	*Interventions:* Both groups received therapy consisting of active, active assisted, and passive range of motion exercises. Use of the sling was discontinued when therapy began. Progressive resistive exercises were initiated if tolerated to increase strength. *Outcome measures:* • Change in active ROM • Change in grip strength • Length of time to return to work with empirical light duty.	In Group 1, 52% of participants did not achieve full active extension, compared with 4% in Group 2. No statistically significant difference was detected in grip strength between the two groups. The average time for return to work was 4 months for Group 1 and 2 months for Group 2. Thus, the sooner the therapy was initiated after surgery, the sooner the participant recovered and achieved full range of motion. The use of modalities may have given temporary relief of symptoms but did not affect the outcome of range of motion.	All participants were treated by the same surgeon and therapist, which may have biased the results. Surgical techniques and therapy procedures may have changed significantly since 1995.	Range of motion exercises should be initiated as soon as 1 day postoperatively to prevent loss of motion and to minimize flexion contractures following cubital tunnel release with medial epicondylectomy.

Reference: Warwick, L., & Seradge, H. (1995). Early versus late range of motion following cubital tunnel surgery. *Journal of Hand Therapy, 8*, 245–248.

Appendix D.
Evidence Table —
Forearm, Wrist, and Hand

Evidence Table—Forearm, Wrist, and Hand

Author/Year	Study Objectives	Level/Design/ Participants	Intervention and Outcome Measures	Results	Study Limitations	Implications for Occupational Therapy
Bleakley, McDonough, & MacAuley, 2004	To assess the evidence base for the use of cryotherapy in treatment of acute soft tissue injuries	I—Systematic review $N = 1,469$ participants (22 trials) recovering from a soft tissue injury or orthopedic surgical intervention and receiving inpatient, outpatient, or home-based cryotherapy	*Interventions:* Participants were treated with inpatient, outpatient, or home-based cryotherapy used in isolation or in combination with other treatments. *Outcome measures:* ■ Objective or subjective reports of pain, swelling, function, or ROM.	Marginal evidence indicates that ice plus exercise is most effective in reducing pain following ankle sprain and surgery. Little evidence indicates that ice added to compression had any effect in hospital inpatient settings. There was no evidence to support an optimal mode or duration of ice application.	The included RCT's scored an average PEDro score of only 3 and 4, indicating that the studies were of low quality. Differences in treatment protocols made it nearly impossible to make comparisons within and among studies. Methodological problems with many studies limit generalizability of the findings.	More research is required to provide evidence-based guidelines for the treatment of acute soft-tissue injuries. Cryotherapy is a commonly used intervention throughout the medical community, but evidence presented in this review for its use is severely limited. Because this study does offer marginal evidence that ice can be effective with pain in postsurgical cases, clinicians who understand the underlying physiology and therapeutic effect expected may continue to use it.

Reference: Bleakley, C., McDonough, S., & MacAuley, D. (2004). The use of ice in the treatment of acute soft-tissue injury: A systematic review of randomized controlled trials. *American Journal of Sports Medicine, 32,* 251–261.

Author/Year	Study Objectives	Level/Design/ Participants	Intervention and Outcome Measures	Results	Study Limitations	Implications for Occupational Therapy
Brosseau et al., 2002	To assess the efficacy of deep transverse friction massage for treating tendinitis.	I—Systematic review $N = 2$ trials for those with clinical diagnosis of tendinitis at knee or elbow	*Interventions:* Deep transverse friction massage was compared to groups receiving placebo treatment, no therapy, or other active treatments. *Outcome measures:* Pain ■ ROM ■ Muscle strength ■ Endurance ■ Functional status.	No evidence was found of clinically important benefits of deep transverse friction massage for treating tendinitis.	The review included only 2 studies.	Although anecdotal reports are plentiful that deep transverse friction massage gives positive results (especially when used with other modalities such as ultrasound, heat, cold, or splinting), this study does not support it as a viable treatment technique. Therapists are therefore encouraged to use this approached only when client benefit can be measured. Further research using randomized trials, validated outcome measures, and high-quality reporting methods is needed.

Reference: Brosseau, L., Casimiro, L., Milne, S., Robinson, V. A., Shea, B. J., Tugwell, P., et al. (2002). Deep transverse friction massage for treating tendonitis. *Cochrane Database of Systematic Reviews, 4,* CD003528.

Brosseau, MacLeay, Robinson, Tugwell, & Wells, 2003	To evaluate the effectiveness of different exercise intensities for people with osteoarthritis	I—Systematic review of comparative controlled studies *N* = 39 participants (1 trial) with osteoarthritis	*Interventions:* Participants engaging in high-intensity and low-intensity aerobic exercise (stationary cycling) were compared with a control group receiving no exercise treatment. *Outcome measures:* ■ Functional status ■ Gait ■ Pain ■ Aerobic capacity.	No significant differences were found between high-intensity and low-intensity exercise in treatment of osteoarthritis of the knee on measures of functional status; both types of exercise resulted in improvements. A trend toward better results was noted for low-intensity exercise vs. no exercise compared with high-intensity exercise vs. no exercise in pain and functional status.	Only one study was included in the review. This study suggests that an occupational therapy practitioner can create an appropriate aerobic activity program that will lead to increased aerobic capacity and decreased pain. Further research is required to establish evidence that the outcome of this type of exercise can be generalized to clients with osteoarthritis of the upper extremity.

Reference: Brosseau, L., MacLeay, L., Robinson, V. A., Tugwell, P., & Wells, G. (2003). Intensity of exercise for the treatment of osteoarthritis. *Cochrane Database of Systematic Reviews, 2,* CD004259.

Brosseau et al., 2004	To assess the effectiveness of low-level laser therapy (LLLT) in the treatment of osteoarthritis	I—Systematic review *N* = 345 participants (7 trials) with osteoarthritis, 184 randomized to LLLT and 161 to placebo laser	*Interventions:* Controlled clinical trials of LLLT for participants with a diagnosis of osteoarthritis were selected for study. *Outcome measures:* ■ Pain reduction ■ ROM.	The results of the review were inconclusive. Three trials showed no effect on pain, two demonstrated beneficial effects, and one found increased knee ROM (lower doses and higher doses yielded same result). Other outcomes for joint tenderness and strength were not significant.	Clinical application of LLLT was heterogeneous, including different dosages, wavelengths, and types of LLLT. There may have been a publication bias in the articles chosen. This review does not offer support for the use of LLLT for osteoarthritic conditions. Further research is needed before the effectiveness of LLLT can be determined.

Reference: Brosseau, L., Robinson, V., Wells, G., deBie, R., Gam, A., Harman, K., et al. (2004). Low level laser therapy (Classes I, II and III) for treating osteoarthritis. *Cochrane Database of Systematic Reviews, 3,* CD002046.

(continued)

Evidence Table—Forearm, Wrist, and Hand (cont.)

Author/Year	Study Objectives	Level/Design/ Participants	Intervention and Outcome Measures	Results	Study Limitations	Implications for Occupational Therapy
Case-Smith, 2003	To measure functional outcomes after outpatient occupational therapy for clients who had an upper extremity injury, surgery, or both To measure the correlation of the Canadian Occupational Performance Measure (COPM) with other outcome measures	III—Descriptive study $N = 37$ participants (4 lost to follow-up) receiving typical hand therapy treatment provided by an occupational therapy practitioner for diagnosis of hand injury within 30 days	*Interventions:* Treatment included physical agent modalities, manual techniques, and therapeutic activities. Clients received a mean of 13 hours of outpatient occupational therapy services; they received no other services at that time. *Outcome measures:* ■ Functional performance gains (COPM; Disabilities of the Arm, Shoulder, and Head [DASH]; SF–36) ■ Community integration (Community Integration Questionnaire).	Functional performance gains following 6–8 weeks of services were significant. The Community Integration Questionnaire, initially created for patients with brain injuries, was found not to be beneficial in this setting.	The relatively small sample size with a combination of diagnoses creates difficulty with generalizing results. Questionnaires were completed by participants, possibly introducing error. The evaluating therapist was not blinded to participant. Treatments varied among participants depending on diagnosis. Treatments were not described beyond the general descriptive categories. There was no control group. Study did not control for variables such as client motivation, attitude, spontaneous recovery, and presence or lack of supportive environment.	Occupational therapists seeking outcome measures that are sensitive to changes following hand therapy intervention may consider use of the COPM, DASH, and SF–36 as pretreatment and posttreatment assessment tools. This study supports occupational interventions as resulting in improved function but does not support any specific intervention or interventions.

Reference: Case-Smith, J. (2003). Outcomes in hand rehabilitation using occupational therapy services. *American Journal of Occupational Therapy, 57,* 499–506.

Author/Year	Study Objectives	Level/Design/ Participants	Intervention and Outcome Measures	Results	Study Limitations	Implications for Occupational Therapy
Egan & Brousseau, 2007	To review the evidence regarding the effectiveness of splinting for carpometacarpal osteoarthritis of the thumb	I—Systematic review of studies of various designs $N = 258$ participants (7 trials)	*Interventions:* Participants were treated with a variety of splints, including prefabricated short neoprene splint, custom-made short opponens thermoplastic splint, short opponens	On average, participants who received a splint obtained some relief from it. No splint was found to be more effective than another for reducing pain and enhancing function.	Internal validity is challenged by the possibility of a placebo effect and fact that other forms of treatment (e.g., nonsteroidal anti-inflammatory drugs) were initiated at same time as the splint.	Evidence suggests some correlation between splinting of the osteoarthritic carpometacarpal joint and decreased pain. Clients for whom splinting diminishes pain can better use the hand to

Author/Year	Objective	Design/Level & Participants	Intervention & Outcome Measures	Results	Implications for Practice
			splint, volar long opponens splint, semirigid orthosis that did not cross wrist, firm elastic splint with semirigid strip along dorsal side of thumb, supple elastic wrist gauntlet, custom-made leather splint, semi-stable textile splint, and no splint. Wear times varied. *Outcome measures:* ■ Pain ■ Function ■ Wearing comfort ■ Pinch strength ■ Desire for surgery.	None of the studies used a design that resulted in strong evidence of effectiveness. The question of overall effectiveness of splinting in providing pain relief remains unanswered by this review.	participate in occupation-based tasks. The therapist may offer a choice of device based on client preference or context; no design was found to be more or less effective than another.

Reference: Egan, M. Y., & Brosseau, L. (2007). Splinting for osteoarthritis of the carpometacarpal joint: A review of the evidence. *American Journal of Occupational Therapy, 61,* 70–78.

Author/Year	Objective	Design/Level & Participants	Intervention & Outcome Measures	Results	Implications for Practice
Feehan & Bassett, 2004	To determine if there is scientifically valid evidence for the effect of early motion (<21 days) on joints surrounding an extra-articular hand fracture on fracture healing or functional outcomes	I—Systematic review of quasi-randomized studies *N* = 459 participants (6 trials) with simple, closed, metacarpal fractures occurring in 2nd through 5th digits	*Interventions:* Studies compared complex postfracture immobilization of both joints proximal and distal to the fracture with motion of one or both joints adjacent to the fracture. Joint motion had to be initiated in the first 21 days after fracture or reduction. *Outcome measures:* ■ Fracture healing status ■ Time to union or malunion (primary measure) ■ Secondary medical and surgical interventions (secondary measure)	Early motion resulted in earlier recovery of mobility and strength and earlier return to work and did not affect fracture alignment. All studies were poor in quality. No study reported use of a standardized measure of time to clinical or boney union or a score on a standardized hand function test or quality of life instrument.	Current evidence does not support or refute the use of early motion of joints surrounding an extra-articular fracture. Further research is warranted. Secondary outcomes of the study support the use of custom-molded fracture braces for metacarpal fractures and appear to support the notion that early movement may be beneficial while causing no harm to the fracture site. Therapists should not use these findings as conclusive because of their limitations.

Evidence Table—Forearm, Wrist, and Hand (cont.)

Author/Year	Study Objectives	Level/Design/ Participants	Intervention and Outcome Measures	Results	Study Limitations	Implications for Occupational Therapy
Feehan & Bassett, 2004 (cont.)			■ Functional status ■ Standardized hand function or health-related quality of life (primary measure) ■ Secondary measures also included functional strength, mobility, pain, satisfaction, ADLs, and IADLs.			

Reference: Feehan, L., & Bassett, K. (2004). Is there evidence for early mobilization following an extraarticular hand fracture? *Journal of Hand Therapy, 17,* 300–308.

Author/Year	Study Objectives	Level/Design/ Participants	Intervention and Outcome Measures	Results	Study Limitations	Implications for Occupational Therapy
Field et al., 2000	To evaluate the effects of massage therapy on reduction of postburn itching and pain and on reduction of anxiety and depressed mood	I—Randomized controlled trial *N* = 20 participants, mean age 38.2 years, randomly assigned to massage therapy (treatment group) or standard care (control group)	*Interventions:* Control group received standard medical care (physician visits, medication, physical therapy or occupational therapy, cocoa butter to closed wounds without massage). Treatment group received massage therapy for 30 min, 2 times per week for 5 weeks). Massage therapists applied mild to moderate pressure with cocoa butter as a lubricant in a stroking manner; pressured movements from perimeter of wound to center using pads of fingers; circular, transverse, and vertical strokes for 10 min; skin rolling; and long strokes.	Treatment group experienced reduced itching, anxiety, depressed mood, and pain. Long-term improvement occurred in all areas from before first treatment day to last treatment day.	Participants were all from low socioeconomic groups; it is unclear if results are generalizable. Standard medical care that was continued by physical therapists or occupational therapists was not fully described. It is unclear if this standard treatment included methods that may have contributed to outcomes.	The preparatory method of massage for hand injury or postsurgical clients can reduce scarring, pain, and edema and increase tissue extensibility. Massage as a treatment method is plausible and supported. This study also points to the positive effects of massage on the psychological status of the client, which can further support goals of participation in daily living and occupations.

Reference: Field, T., Peck, M., Hernandez-Reif, M., Krugman, S., Burman, I., & Ozment-Schenck, L. (2000). Postburn itching, pain, and psychological symptoms are reduced with massage therapy. *Journal of Burn Care and Rehabilitation, 21,* 189–193.

Author/Year	Purpose	Design/Sample	Interventions	Results	Limitations/Comments
			Outcome measures: ■ Itching severity (based on Present Pain Intensity Scale of the Short Form McGill Pain Questionnaire) ■ Pain (Visual Analog Scale, McGill Pain Questionnaire) ■ Anxiety and depressed mood (State Trait Anxiety Inventory, Profile of Mood States).		
Guzelkucuk, Duman, Taskaynatan, & Dincer, 2007	To compare the efficacy of therapeutic activities that simulate ADLs with traditional therapeutic exercises in the management of injured hands in young adult patients	I—Randomized controlled trial *N* = 36 participants with functional hand loss due to injury; 20 allocated to the treatment group, 16 to the control group, average age 23 years, average time between injury or surgery and therapy 102 days	*Interventions:* Control group was provided with an appropriate twice-daily treatment program comprising passive, active assistive, active ROM, and strengthening activities. In addition, physical agent modalities were applied. Treatment group received the same intervention as the control group for one session per day, with a second session comprising 25 activities that simulated ADLs. Treatment continued for 3 weeks, 5 days per week. Participants were discharged to a home program.	Both groups had improved at 2-month follow-up, but the treatment group experienced significantly greater improvements (including functional outcomes), except for total ROM and abduction.	Study was not blind. Compliance with the home program was not assessed. Chronic and acute conditions were included in both groups. Efficacy of activities with specific types of injuries was not determined. Sample size was small. This study provides evidence that naturalized use of the hand in meaningful and relevant activities combining multiple movement patterns, use of force, and volition is a more effective treatment option than straight exercise alone.

(continued)

Evidence Table—Forearm, Wrist, and Hand (cont.)

Author/Year	Study Objectives	Level/Design/ Participants	Intervention and Outcome Measures	Results	Study Limitations	Implications for Occupational Therapy
Guzelkucuk, Duman, Taskaynatan, & Dincer, 2007 (cont.)			*Outcome measures:* ■ Grip strength ■ Pinch strength ■ Finger pulp–distal palmar crease distance ■ Total active movement ■ Range of opposition ■ Range of abduction ■ Hand function (Jebson hand function test; Disabilities of Arm, Shoulder, and Hand).			

Reference: Guzelkucuk, U., Duman, I., Taskaynatan, M., & Dincer, K. (2007). Comparison of therapeutic activities with therapeutic exercises in the rehabilitation of young adult patients with hand injuries. *Journal of Hand Surgery, 32,* 1429–1435.

Author/Year	Study Objectives	Level/Design/ Participants	Intervention and Outcome Measures	Results	Study Limitations	Implications for Occupational Therapy
Haythornthwaite, Lawrence, & Fauerbach, 2001	To test the efficacy of two brief cognitive interventions in supplementing regular medical treatment for pain during dressing change	I—Randomized controlled study *N* = 42 adult participants with 2nd- and 3rd-degree burns covering 3%–65% of total body surface area Participants were randomly assigned to one of three groups—sensory focusing, distraction, or control.	*Interventions:* Before the morning dressing change, participants listened to 20-min audiotapes that taught them how to use the coping strategy. Participants in the sensory focusing group were instructed to focus on the present moment and not to anticipate pain. Participants in the distraction group were instructed to listen to and focus on music of their choice. They were repeatedly prompted to practice the technique during the 4-stage dressing change. The control group received no intervention.	Sensory focusing resulted in higher ratings of relief, whereas distraction, which included self-selected music and music appreciation training, did not show any beneficial effects. Sensory focusing also changed the memory of painful procedures, supporting its utility for multiple painful procedures.	The methodology, which required participants to record pain at 10-min intervals, may have interfered with the intervention. Sample size was relatively small. Nursing procedures, timing, and duration of dressing changes varied.	This study supports that notion that instructing the client in the coping strategy of sensory focusing may be beneficial in reducing the experience of pain during treatment. Occupational therapists can easily and cost-effectively incorporate these strategies into treatment sessions to improve the quality of the client experience.

Outcome measures:
- Pain
- Degree of relief
- Satisfaction
- Depression
- Analgesic medication use.

Reference: Haythornthwaite, J., Lawrence, J. W., & Fauerbach, J. A. (2001). Brief cognitive interventions for burn pain. *Annals of Behavioral Medicine, 23,* 42–49.

| Karjalainen et al., 2000 | To determine the effectiveness of biopsychosocial rehabilitation for upper limb repetitive strain injuries among working age adults | I—Systematic review of randomized controlled trials and prospective, concurrent controlled trials

N = 80 (2 trials) for those ages 18–65 years with diagnosis of repetitive strain injury participating in a biopsychosocial rehabilitation program | *Interventions:*
Studies examined outcomes for inpatient or outpatient biopsychosocial programs that included a physician consultation plus a psychological, social, or vocational intervention or a combination.

Outcome Measures:
- Pain intensity (Visual Analog Scale, ordinal scale)
- Global status (overall improvement)
- Disorder-specific functional status (Upper Extremity Function Scale [UEFS], Neck and Upper Limb Index [NULI])
- Generic functional status or quality of life (Disabilities of the Arm, Shoulder and Hand [DASH], West Haven-Yale Multidimensional Pain Inventory [WHYMPI]). | There was little scientific evidence for the effectiveness of biopsychosocial rehabilitation on repetitive strain injuries.

Only two studies were included, both of low quality. | This review does not support biopsychosocial rehabilitation for repetitive strain injuries. Further research in this area is strongly recommended before conclusions can be drawn about the potential effects of this approach. |

(continued)

Evidence Table—Forearm, Wrist, and Hand (cont.)

Author/Year	Study Objectives	Level/Design/ Participants	Intervention and Outcome Measures	Results	Study Limitations	Implications for Occupational Therapy
Karjalainen et al., 2000 *(cont.)*			• Ability to work • Health care consumption and cost • Satisfaction with treatment.			

Reference: Karjalainen, K., Malmivaara, A., van Tulder, M., Roine, R., Jauhiainen, M., Hurri, H., et al. (2000). Biopsychosocial rehabilitation for upper limb repetitive strain injuries in working age adults. *Cochrane Database of Systematic Reviews, 3*, CD002269.

Author/Year	Study Objectives	Level/Design/ Participants	Intervention and Outcome Measures	Results	Study Limitations	Implications for Occupational Therapy
Michlovitz, Harris, & Watkins, 2004	To investigate the effectiveness of nonsurgical interventions to restore ROM in participants who have sustained fracture, fracture and dislocation, joint injury, and other soft tissue injuries	I—Systematic review including randomized controlled or quasi-randomized controlled trials, cohort study, case series, and case report. *N* = 26 trials included in the review	*Interventions:* Nine articles dealt with splinting and casting, six with joint mobilization, two with continuous passive motion, two with injection, two with injection vs. other therapy, four with exercise, and three with in-clinic versus home exercise. No articles described heat modalities. *Outcome measures:* • ROM • Pain • Functional status • Activities of daily living • Length of treatment • Return to activity • Participant satisfaction.	Consistent evidence suggests positive effectiveness of splints to increase joint ROM. Moderate support exists for joint mobilization techniques for those with joint stiffness. Some studies indicate that continuous passive motion may be a viable alternative to ROM exercise in selected postoperative cases, but there is very little literature on this expensive and time-consuming method. Four studies supported passive ROM as an intervention to increase motion in stiff joints. Both home- and clinic-based treatment approaches were viable. Faster gains in shoulder ROM were realized following a steroid injection.	Articles were of moderate to low quality. There was no consistent approach to splinting between articles. The impact of ROM on disability was not described.	Evidence presented supports the use of commonly used interventions such as splinting, joint mobilization, exercise, and home exercise programs. Continuous passive motion units were minimally supported as beneficial in limited cases; they are not a standard treatment at this time. Occupational therapy practitioners can recommend steroid injections to the physician if they feel this method of increasing ROM is in the best interest of the client.

Reference: Michlovitz, S., Harris, B., & Watkins, M. (2004). Therapy interventions for improving joint range of motion: A systematic review. *Journal of Hand Therapy, 17*, 118–131.

| Michlovitz, Hun, Erasala, Hengehold, & Weingand, 2004 | To evaluate the efficacy of continuous low-level heat wrap therapy for the treatment of various sources of wrist pain, including strain and sprain, tendinosis, osteoarthritis, and carpal tunnel syndrome (CTS).

To evaluate the efficacy of continuous low-level heat wrap as compared with oral placebo | I—Prospective, randomized, parallel, single-blind (investigator), placebo-controlled, multicenter trial

N = 94 participants (1 lost at follow-up) in general good health with wrist pain following surgical intervention <6 months previously | *Interventions:*
Participants with moderate or greater wrist pain were randomized and stratified to receive efficacy evaluation (heat wrap, oral placebo) or blinding (oral acetaminophen, unheated wrap).

Outcome measures:
■ Pain (pain relief scale, 0–5)
■ Joint stiffness (10-point numerical rating scale)
■ Grip strength (dynamometer)
■ Perceived pain and disability (Patient-Rated Wrist Evaluation)
■ Symptom severity and functional status for participants with carpal tunnel syndrome (Symptom Severity Scale and Functional Status Scale). | Continuous low-level heat wrap therapy was effective in the treatment of common conditions causing wrist pain and impairment. Heat wrap provided greater pain relief and joint stiffness reduction than placebo.

The heat wrap group demonstrated significantly improved grip strength over the placebo group in the short term but not at follow-up. The carpal tunnel group showed significant improvement in grip strength during the study and at follow-up.

Differences in pain and disability were not significant between participants with osteoarthritis, tendinosis, and strain or sprain. For those with CTS, change was significant for heat wrap group. | Study is of good quality. | This study supports the use of low-level heat wraps as part of a home program to enhance the ability of clients to engage in ADL and work and leisure pursuits. Low-level prolonged heat wraps can reduce pain and stiffness within the clinic during treatment sessions to enhance client tolerance and participation in functional activities. Further research is required to establish the long-term effects of these methods of improving motion, reducing pain, and enhancing occupational performance. |

Reference: Michlovitz, S., Hun, L., Erasala, G. N., Hengehold, D. A., & Weingand, K. W. (2004). Continuous low-level heat wrap therapy is effective for treating wrist pain. *Archives of Physical Medicine Rehabilitation, 85*, 1409–1416.

(continued)

Evidence Table—Forearm, Wrist, and Hand (cont.)

Author/Year	Study Objectives	Level/Design/ Participants	Intervention and Outcome Measures	Results	Study Limitations	Implications for Occupational Therapy
Muller et al., 2004	To determine the effectiveness of hand therapy interventions for carpal tunnel syndrome (CTS)	I—Systematic review *N* = 24 trials	*Interventions:* Participants were treated with a variety of interventions, including splinting, ultrasound, nerve gliding exercises, yoga, low-level laser therapy, magnetic therapy, manual therapy, acupuncture, and combined therapies. *Outcome measures:* ■ General symptomology ■ Severity of pain ■ Sleep ■ Nerve conduction studies ■ Numbness and tingling ■ Morning stiffness ■ Paresthesias ■ Tactile sensation ■ Pinch and grip strength.	Splinting was supported by five studies; various types of splints and various angles were found effective. Twenty 15-min treatments of deep, pulsed ultrasound decreased symptoms, reduced sensory loss, and improved median nerve conduction and strength. Ten treatments of superficial, continuous ultrasound for 5 min were not effective. Nerve gliding exercises reduced pain and increased ROM compared with no treatment. One session of brief magnetic therapy did not decrease pain more than sham treatment; both decreased pain. Prolonged therapy in wrist support wraps improved symptoms of numbness and tingling and improved nerve conduction studies more than sham treatment. Laser therapy was supported only by one Level IV study. Biweekly 60–90-min hatha yoga sessions for 8 weeks improved symptoms but did not improve grip strength	Articles not published in English were not used, hand searches were not conducted, and authors of articles were not contacted to determine availability of more current research. Magnetic treatment that used splints may have been limited by effect of splint use on holding magnets in place; splints alone have been found to be effective. Manual therapy results depended on the particular techniques being used.	Both custom splints and prefabricated splints are effective, as are a variety of angles of immobilization. Regarding ultrasound treatment, therapists should consider parameters that include pulsed treatment of lower frequency vs. more superficial treatments of a continuous nature, as well as number and length of treatment. Nerve gliding exercises were shown to be effective. Manual therapy may be considered an effective preparatory method by occupational therapists versed in the technique. Low-level laser therapy and acupuncture were not strongly supported by this review and are not currently used in occupational therapy standard protocols. Yoga is a complementary intervention (vs. approach) that occupational therapists may recommend to a client as an adjunct to intervention to relieve pain symptoms. Yoga would require additional training on the part of the occupational therapy practitioner for safe

			or decrease pain more than splinting alone. Manual therapy (carpal tunnel mobilization combined with flexor retinaculum stretch) effectively relieved pain, but carpal tunnel maneuver with stretches of digits 3 and 4 did not change nerve conduction.		and effective administration.
			Evidence supporting acupuncture as a treatment for CTS is limited; no conclusion was drawn in this review.		

Reference: Muller, M., Tsui, D., Schnurr, R., Biddulph-Deisroth, L., Hard, J., & MacDermid, J. C. (2004). Effectiveness of hand therapy interventions in primary management of carpal tunnel syndrome: A systematic review. *Journal of Hand Therapy, 17,* 210–228.

Nash, Mickan, Del Mar, & Glaziou, 2004	To determine if benefit or harm comes from mobilizing or immobilizing an acute limb injury in adults	I—Systematic review *N* = 3,366 participants (49 trials) treated with immobilization for soft tissue injuries and fractures of both upper and lower limbs	*Interventions:* Studies were divided into 4 groups: lower limb fractures, other lower limb injury, upper limb fractures, and other upper limb injuries. Groups were further divided into trials using limb support versus no support. *Outcome measures:* ■ Patient-centered outcomes ■ Functional outcomes ■ Measures of global function including subjective and objective criteria such as pain, stiffness, swelling, use of supports, stair climbing,	All studies reported either no difference between rest and early mobilization protocols or benefits from early mobilization. Benefits included earlier return to work; decreased pain, swelling, and stiffness; and greater preserved ROM. Early mobilization caused no increase in deformity, complications, or residual symptoms. The reviewers did not contact authors for clarification or updated research. Many studies were of poor quality; review focused discussion on studies of higher quality only. The reviewers did not list all diagnoses included in all studies; it is not known if acute tendon repairs, nerve injuries, or joint replacements (as examples) were present in the early mobilization group.	This research suggests that movement, compared with rest, will not harm an acute soft tissue injury, supporting interventions that encourage occupational engagement. Therapists are cautioned against using this review as a general guideline, as many upper extremity injuries do require a period of protected movement. All treatment approaches to acute injuries should be done under the guidance of a physician.

(continued)

Evidence Table—Forearm, Wrist, and Hand (cont.)

Author/Year	Study Objectives	Level/Design/ Participants	Intervention and Outcome Measures	Results	Study Limitations	Implications for Occupational Therapy
Nash, Mickan, Del Mar, & Glaziou, 2004 (cont.)			work, sport playing, and ADL ■ Range of motion ■ Deformity and other complications ■ Participant preference.			be done under the guidance of a physician.

Reference: Nash, C. E., Mickan, M., Del Mar, C. B., & Glasziou, P. P. (2004). Resting injured limbs delays recovery: A systematic review. *Journal of Family Practice, 53,* 706–712.

Author/Year	Study Objectives	Level/Design/ Participants	Intervention and Outcome Measures	Results	Study Limitations	Implications for Occupational Therapy
O'Brien & Pandit, 2006	To determine the effect of silicone gel sheeting for prevention or treatment of hypertrophic or keloid scarring in newly healed wounds and those with established scars	I—Systematic review *N* = 559 participants (13 trials) ages 2–81 years	*Interventions:* Trials compared adhesive silicone gel sheeting with a control, such as nonsilicon gel sheeting, silicone gel plates with added vitamin E, laser therapy, triamcinolone acetonide injection, or nonadhesive silicone gel sheeting. *Outcome measures:* (prevention studies): ■ Number of people who developed scarring as determined by blood flow, hyperpigmentation, erythema, scar thickness, and regularity of scar *Outcome measures:* (treatment studies): ■ Change in scar size (area, length, volume, height, or width) measured with ruler, impression, or ultrasound.	Prevention interventions, when compared to no treatment, reduced the incidence of hypertrophic scarring. Gel sheeting increased scar elasticity in established scarring.	The reviewers considered both the prevention and the correction studies to be highly susceptible to bias and of poor quality.	Silicone gel sheeting is supported as a preparatory method; occupational therapists using gel sheets should exercise caution and note the limitations of this study.

Reference: O'Brien, L., & Pandit, A. (2006). Silicon gel sheeting for preventing and treating hypertrophic and keloid scars. *Cochrane Database of Systematic Reviews, 1,* CD003826.

Author/Year	Study Objectives	Level/Design/Participants	Intervention and Outcome Measures	Results	Study Limitations
O'Connor, Marshall, & Massy-Westropp, 2003	To evaluate the effectiveness of nonsurgical treatment (other than steroid injection) for carpal tunnel syndrome vs. a placebo or other nonsurgical (control) interventions in improving clinical outcomes	I—Systematic review of randomized and quasi-randomized studies N = 884 participants (21 trials) with a diagnosis of nonsurgical release carpal tunnel syndrome	*Interventions:* Treatment methods included splinting, ultrasound, yoga, carpal tunnel mobilization, ergonomic keyboards, magnet therapy, laser acupuncture, exercise, and chiropractic care. Only steroid injection treatment was excluded. *Outcome measures:* ■ Clinical symptoms (pain and paresthesias) ■ Function ■ Quality of life.	Moderate evidence indicates short-term benefit from oral steroids; limited evidence suggests that splinting, ultrasound, yoga, and carpal bone mobilization can be effective. Equivocal results were noted for the use of ergonomic keyboards to reduce pain and improve function. Other nonsurgical techniques (magnet therapy, nerve gliding, and chiropractic) were not found to be effective.	Several studies had high levels of bias.	Occupational therapy treatment for carpal tunnel syndrome typically includes splinting and often includes ultrasound and mobilization techniques (in addition to others). Although limited, these studies support continued use of these methods by occupational therapy practitioners. Further investigation is warranted.

Reference: O'Connor, D., Marshall, S., & Massy-Westropp, N. (2003). Non-surgical treatment (other than steroid injection) for carpal tunnel syndrome. *Cochrane Database of Systematic Reviews, 1,* CD003219.

Author/Year	Study Objectives	Level/Design/Participants	Intervention and Outcome Measures	Results	Study Limitations
Oerlemans, Goris, de Boo, & Oostendorp, 1999	To determine the influence of various treatments on the severity of permanent impairment of those with reflex sympathetic dystrophy	I—Prospective, randomized controlled, single-blind clinical trial N = 135 participants with an average of 3.6 months of reflex sympathetic dystrophy symptoms in one upper extremity Participants were randomly assigned to a physical therapy or occupational therapy group and a control group that received social work services.	*Interventions:* Participants underwent 30 min of treatment per session consisting of methods and techniques outlined in a treatment protocol. The occupational therapy protocol included reduction of inflammation, normalization of sensation, functional activities, and ADL retraining. Main objectives of physical therapy were to increase pain control, extinguish source of pain, and improve skills. *Outcome measures:* ■ Impairment ratings (American Medical Association's *Guides to the Evalu-*	After the 12-month study period, no significant differences in impairment ratings were detected between the treatment groups and the control group or within the treatment groups themselves.	Areas measured as impairments may not reflect treatment offered by therapies. Participants whose symptoms were longstanding may already have reached a natural plateau. The subjective experience of participants was not taken into account; the impairment rating did not measure actual functional disability. Participants were able to switch groups on request. Standard physical therapy and occupational therapy treatment pro-	The limitations of this study and differences between Dutch and U.S. protocols limit the applicability of findings. A similar study using a protocol design more in keeping with common practice in the United States might provide more useful results.

(continued)

Evidence Table—Forearm, Wrist, and Hand (cont.)

Author/Year	Study Objectives	Level/Design/ Participants	Intervention and Outcome Measures	Results	Study Limitations	Implications for Occupational Therapy
Oerlemans, Goris, de Boo, & Oostendorp, 1999 (cont.)			*ation of Permanent Impairment)* ■ Joint ROM ■ Grip strength ■ 2-point discrimination.		tocols in the Netherlands may not be representative of treatment approaches used by U.S. therapists (particularly occupational therapists).	

Reference: Oerlemans, H. M. Goris, R. J. A., de Boo, T., & Oostendorp, R. A. (1999). Do physical therapy and occupational therapy reduce the impairment percentage in reflex sympathetic dystrophy? *American Journal of Physical Medicine and Rehabilitation, 78,* 533–539.

Author/Year	Study Objectives	Level/Design/ Participants	Intervention and Outcome Measures	Results	Study Limitations	Implications for Occupational Therapy
Oud, Beelen, Eijffinger & Nollet, 2007	To systematically review available evidence for the effectiveness of sensory reeducation to improve the sensibility of the hand in persons with a peripheral nerve injury of the upper limb	I—Systematic review of randomized controlled trials, nonrandomized controlled trials, and experiments without a control group (before–after design) *N* = 274 (7 trials)	*Interventions:* Interventions included rotating tactile stimulation discs, pocket-size tactile stimulator, familiar objects with different shapes and textures, and early- and late-phase sensory stimulation. *Outcome measures:* ■ Moving 2-point discrimination ■ Constant 2-point discrimination ■ Cutaneous pressure threshold.	There was limited evidence for the effectiveness of sensory reeducation; statistically significant improvement occurred in only one high-quality randomized controlled trial.	Five of the studies included in the review were of poor methodological quality.	This systematic review yields little support for the preparatory approach of sensory reeducation when treating clients with peripheral nerve injury. To enhance occupational engagement that may be impaired by diminished sensation and to ensure client safety, practitioners should choose a compensatory approach to treatment. Additional studies are required to provide evidence that supports improved safe and successful engagement in occupations using compensatory techniques.

Reference: Oud, T., Beelen, A., Eijffinger, E., & Nollet, F. (2007). Sensory re-education after nerve injury of the upper limb: A systematic review. *Clinical Rehabilitation, 21,* 483–494.

Richard, Miller, Finley, & Jones, 1987	To investigate two common interventions for increasing finger flexion ROM—passive exercise and static wrapping	I—Randomized controlled trial *N* = 6 participants with combined full- and partial-thickness dorsal hand burns	*Intervention:* The therapist administered passive ROM exercise to involved finger joints except distal interphalangeal joint for 10 min and wrapped affected joints in full mitten configuration using 3-in elastic bandage; wrap was left in place 10 min. Thirteen trials were performed of each technique; time frame was not reported. *Outcome measures:* ■ Active ROM (tool not explicitly stated).	Passive exercise was more effective in increasing metacarpophalangeal joint flexion. Static wrapping was better at increasing proximal interphalangeal joint flexion.	Sample size was small and intervention period was brief.	Evidence supports the use of both manual passive exercise and wrapping as preparatory techniques in hand clinics. In the case of bilateral hand burns, it is recommended that the more involved hand be wrapped while the less involved hand is exercised. Further research is required to establish the validity of the outcomes and long-term effects of these methods. It remains unclear whether the gains in ROM realized actually translated into an improvement in occupational performance.

Reference: Richard, R. L., Miller, S. F., Finley, R. K., & Jones, L. M. (1987). Comparison of the effect of passive exercise v. static wrapping on finger range of motion in the burned hand. *Journal of Burn Care and Rehabilitation, 8,* 576–578.

Severens et al., 1999	To study from a societal viewpoint the cost-effectiveness of adjunctive treatment for patients with reflex sympathetic dystrophy of one extremity	I—Randomized controlled trial *N* = 135 participants with diagnosis of reflex sympathetic dystrophy in one upper extremity who experienced symptoms for <1 year Participants were randomly assigned to a physical therapy or occupational therapy group and a control	*Interventions:* Treatments were provided according to preestablished protocols. Participants kept dairies for 2 weeks between follow-up visits to the hospital, which occurred four times during the study. They recorded visits to therapy and other venues regarding their reflex sympathetic dystrophy and money	Only the ISS measures showed a difference between physical therapy vs. occupational therapy and control treatment. Physical therapy and occupational therapy were more costly than the control therapy, but medical costs were similar across groups. Physical therapy was found to result in clini-	Functional abilities and disability were not measured. The cost of occupational therapy, physical therapy, and medical care in the Netherlands may not be comparable to that in the United States. Protocols used and frequencies and durations of treatments provided	The limitations of this study and differences between Dutch and U.S. protocols and costs of therapy, medical supplies, and lost productivity limit the applicability of findings. A similar study using a protocol design more in keeping with common practice in the United States might provide more useful results. *(continued)*

Evidence Table—Forearm, Wrist, and Hand (cont.)

Author/Year	Study Objectives	Level/Design/Participants	Intervention and Outcome Measures	Results	Study Limitations	Implications for Occupational Therapy
Severens et al., 1999 (cont.)		group that received social work services.	spent on medications and supplies related to the condition. *Outcome measures:* ▪ Time missed from work ▪ Pain, edema, skin temperature, and active ROM (Impairment-level Sum Score [ISS]) ▪ Ability to move light objects within 15 sec (modified Greentest) ▪ General health (Sickness Impact Profile) ▪ Money spent on medications and supplies.	ically relevant improvement in reflex sympathetic dystrophy symptoms. Incremental cost-effectiveness ratios indicated that physical therapy was more cost-effective and less costly than occupational therapy and control treatment.	were not described. Standard treatment protocols in the Netherlands may not be representative of those used by U.S. therapists. Participants were able to switch groups.	

Reference: Severens, J. L., Oerlemans, H. M., Weegels, A. J. P. G., van't Hof, M. A., Oostendorp, R. A. B., & Goris, R. J. A. (1999). Cost-effectiveness analysis of adjuvant physical or occupational therapy for patients with reflex sympathetic dystrophy. *Archives of Physical Medicine Rehabilitation, 80,* 1038–1043.

Author/Year	Study Objectives	Level/Design/Participants	Intervention and Outcome Measures	Results	Study Limitations	Implications for Occupational Therapy
van der Windt et al., 1999	To evaluate the effectiveness of ultrasound therapy in the treatment of musculoskeletal disorders	I—Systematic review *N* = 38 trials	*Interventions:* One group received active ultrasound, and the other received either no treatment or placebo control. *Outcomes:* ▪ General improvement (participant report) ▪ Pain (Visual Analog Scale, ordinal scale, pain questionnaire) ▪ Functional disability ▪ ROM.	Little evidence was found to support the use of ultrasound therapy in the treatment of musculoskeletal disorders. Statistical pooling for placebo-controlled trials on lateral epicondylitis yielded results (difference in success rate of 15%, 95% confidence interval 8%–38%) that warrant further investigation.	Publication bias was possible, as only published trial reports were used in review.	Despite anecdotal reports of client benefit from ultrasound, this review did not find clinically important or statistically significant differences in placebo vs. treatment groups in favor of ultrasound. Further investigations into the effects of this modality are warranted. Due to limited support for use of ultrasound, therapists are cautioned to use this modality only when client benefit can be measured.

Reference: van der Windt, D. A., van der Heijden, G. J., van den Berg, S. G., ter Riet, G., de Winter, A. F., & Bouter, L. M. (1999). Ultrasound therapy for musculoskeletal disorders: A systematic review. *Pain, 81,* 257–271.

| Verhagen et al., 2006 | To determine if conservative interventions have a significant impact on short- and long-term outcomes for upper extremity work-related musculoskeletal disorders | I—Systematic review of randomized controlled trials and controlled clinical trials

N = 925 participants (15 trials) with upper extremity work-related musculoskeletal disorders | *Interventions:*
Treatments included exercises, manual therapy, massage, ergonomics, multidisciplinary treatment, splint, and individual and group therapy.

Outcome measures:
■ Pain intensity (Visual Analog Scale, ordinal scale)
■ Global status (overall improvement)
■ Disorder-specific functional status (UEFS, NULI)
■ Generic functional status or quality of life (DASH, WHYMPI)
■ Ability to work
■ Health care consumption and cost
■ Recurrence of injury. | The review found limited evidence for the effectiveness of keyboards with key force displacement or alternate geometry. There was also limited evidence for the effectiveness of individual exercise. The benefit of ergonomic modifications in the workplace was not demonstrated. | The possibility of selection bias exists. The overall quality of studies was poor. A wide range of interventions was examined. No definition was provided of work-relatedness. | This review provides very limited support for the use of ergonomic keyboards and individual exercise. Therapists are therefore cautioned to use these approaches only when client benefit can be measured. |

Reference: Verhagen, A. P., Karels, C., Bierma-Zeinstra, S. M. A., Burdorf, L., Feleus, A., Dahaghin, S., et al. (2006). Ergonomic and physiotherapeutic interventions for treating work-related complaints of the arm, neck or shoulder in adults. *Cochrane Database of Systematic Reviews, 3,* CD003471.

(continued)

Evidence Table—Forearm, Wrist, and Hand (cont.)

Author/Year	Study Objectives	Level/Design/ Participants	Intervention and Outcome Measures	Results	Study Limitations	Implications for Occupational Therapy
Wajon & Ada, 2005	To compare the effects of two 6-week splint and exercise regimens for patients with trapeziometacarpal osteoarthritis	I—Randomized controlled trial *N* = 40 participants with pain at the base of the thumb and diagnosis of Stage I–III trapeziometacarpal osteoarthritis	*Interventions:* The experimental group was taught an abduction exercise routine and given a newly created thumb splint known as the "thumb strap splint." The splint was designed to prevent flexion and adduction of the metacarpal, dorsoradial subluxation of the base of the first metacarpal, and metacarpophalangeal hyperextension. The control group was instructed to wear a short opponens splint. Both groups were instructed to wear the splints full-time (removal for hygiene only) for 2 weeks. For weeks 2–6, splinting continued with the addition of the exercise regimen. For the experimental group, the exercises consisted of pain-free abduction exercise only; the control group's typical treatment program included pain-free pinching exercises with a soft foam block. *Outcome measures:* ■ Pain ■ Strength ■ Hand function.	There was no difference between groups after the 2-week splint program and no difference in pain, strength, or hand function after the 4-week exercise and splint program (weeks 2–6). Both groups improved significantly in all three outcomes measured.	Factors other than the interventions may have accounted for the significant improvements, such as the Hawthorne effect, the placebo effect, and the method of statistical regression.	Because no difference was noted in improvements between the two splints and two pain-free exercise regimens, occupational therapists may freely allow client performance and habits to influence splint and exercise selection (leading to a client-centered approach to treatment).

Reference: Wajon, A., & Ada, L. (2005). No difference between two splint and exercise regimens for people with osteoarthritis of the thumb: A randomized controlled trial. *Australian Journal of Physiotherapy, 51,* 245–249.

Weinstock-Zlotnick, Torres-Gray, & Segal, 2004	To compare the effects of pressure garment work gloves (PGWGs) with sueded palm and standard pressure garment gloves (SPGGs) on functional hand use in individuals with hand burns	III—Quasi-experimental, nonrandomized, repeated measure design *N* = 2 participants with 3 burned hands. PGWG served as the experimental condition, SPGG served as the control condition, and each participating hand was its own control.	*Interventions:* Participants wore one SPGG and one PGWG for 1 week to acclimate to fit and use. Outcomes were measured at the home of the participant; testing was separated by a period of 1 or 2 weeks to decrease the likelihood of training effect. *Outcome measures:* ■ Grip strength (Jamar dynamometer) ■ Pinch meter ■ Sensation (Moberg Pickup Test) ■ Hand function (Jebson–Taylor Hand Function Test) ■ Ease of performance of several ADL skills (Likert-scale rating) ■ Glove preference (Likert-scale rating).	The three participating hands scored better in the PGWG condition than in the SPGG condition in picking up small objects, stacking checkers, picking up heavy objects, zipping, opening and closing a jar, and handling money. Two of the three hands also scored better with the PGWG in picking up light objects with vision intact, opening and closing toothpaste, turning doorknob, and key in lock. One of the three PGWG hands scored better in grip strength, simulated page turning, and simulated feeding with vision occluded. The work glove was unanimously preferred and described as the ideal choice if only one glove was to be allocated. Changes in functional hand use were significant.	Sample size was small; convenience sample may not be appropriately generalized to larger populations. Likert scale used for rating ADL abilities relied on memory of task difficulty, not on actual task performance. Likert scale may not have been a sensitive measure.	Although limited by sample size and outcome measures, the finding of this study that participants had a preference for one glove supports a client-centered approach to equipment provision. Clients should be offered the opportunity to choose gloves that they find improve their functional abilities within desired life tasks.

Reference: Weinstock-Zlotnick, G., Torres-Gray, D., & Segal, R. (2004). Effect of pressure garment work gloves on hand function in patients with hand burns: A pilot study. *Journal of Hand Therapy, 17,* 368–376.

(continued)

Evidence Table—Forearm, Wrist, and Hand *(cont.)*

Author/Year	Study Objectives	Level/Design/ Participants	Intervention and Outcome Measures	Results	Study Limitations	Implications for Occupational Therapy
Werner, Franzblau, & Gell, 2005	To determine if night splinting of workers with carpal tunnel syndrome (CTS) would improve symptoms and median nerve function and affect medical care	I—Randomized controlled trial *N* = 112 auto workers reporting symptoms of CTS	*Interventions:* Both groups (treatment *n* = 63; control *n* = 49) were given instructions in how to reduce ergonomic stressors in both work and home environments via a 20-min video. The treatment group was fitted with a custom hand–wrist orthotic that placed the wrist in neutral position. The most symptomatic hand was chosen for study in participants with bilateral hand involvement. Splints were worn at night for 6 weeks. *Outcome measures:* ■ Validated CTS symptom severity scale ■ 30-day worst-discomfort rating (10-point Visual Analog Scale) ■ Nerve conduction testing.	Splinting reduced discomfort scores for 12 months but produced no difference in symptom severity scale scores. Both groups improved over time, but improvements were greater in the treatment group. No difference in nerve conduction studies was shown between the two groups between pre- and poststudy.	Participants were not blinded to their treatment, and the primary outcome measure was a self-reported questionnaire. Participants were not fully evaluated at 3-month and 6-month intervals. Statistical methodology and loss of participants may have confounded the analysis in the logistic model. Median nerve symptoms in the control group were found to be more severe than in the treatment group, despite randomization.	This study supports (with limitations) splinting the wrist of clients with CTS in neutral position at night and providing education about ergonomics.

Reference: Werner, R. A., Franzblau, A., & Gell, N. (2005). Randomized controlled trial of nocturnal splinting for active workers with symptoms of carpal tunnel syndrome. *Archives of Physical Medicine and Rehabilitation, 86,* 1–7.

Author/Year	Study Objectives	Level/Design/Participants	Intervention and Outcome Measures	Results	Study Limitations	Implications for Occupational Therapy
Wessel, 2004	To evaluate the efficacy of hand exercises for persons with rheumatoid arthritis	I—Systematic review of comparative trials and case studies N = 402 (9 trials)	*Interventions:* Interventions included any form of hand exercise, such as ROM, strengthening, endurance exercises, or motor control or re-learning. Interventions could include a combination of exercise and other modalities. *Outcome measures:* ■ Strength ■ ROM ■ Dexterity ■ Pain ■ Stiffness ■ Self-report of function.	Results for or against the value of hand exercise in the treatment of rheumatoid arthritis are not conclusive, although there is weak evidence that appropriate exercises might lead to long-term strength changes and very short-term changes in stiffness. In general, meta-analysis was not possible because of the wide range of study designs and outcome measures.	Studies used in the review were of low quality. Studies used did not mention expected change that would be considered clinically important. Studies lacked power calculations. Little attempt was made across studies to blind or provide placebo intervention to participants. Studies did not highlight a specific form of intervention.	Inconclusive evidence from this review suggests long-term strength benefits and short-term mobility benefits with exercises that target these areas. Therapists must use clinical reasoning skills combined with knowledge of the pathodynamics of rheumatoid arthritis and the use and effects of exercise when determining if a particular method should be used with a particular client.

Reference: Wessel, J. (2004). The effectiveness of hand exercises for persons with rheumatoid arthritis: A systematic review. *Journal of Hand Therapy, 17,* 174–180.

Author/Year	Study Objectives	Level/Design/Participants	Intervention and Outcome Measures	Results	Study Limitations	Implications for Occupational Therapy
Williams, Westmorland, Schmuck, & MacDermid, 2004	To evaluate the available evidence on workplace rehabilitation interventions for work-related upper extremity disorders	I—Systematic review N = 751 (8 trials) for those receiving workplace-based interventions for upper extremity disorders	*Interventions:* Workplace interventions included ergonomic modifications to the workplace to decrease repetitiveness, force, and awkward positioning and job accommodations such as modified work, light duty work trials, and graded return to work. *Outcome measures:* ■ Pain (Visual Analog Scale) ■ Pre- and post-electromyography testing	The evidence is insufficient to identify effective workplace rehabilitation interventions for work-related upper extremity disorders.	Studies were limited by small sample sizes, lack of standardized outcome measures, and inadequate reporting of interventions and results.	Evidence has not been established that supports workplace interventions for work-related upper extremity disorders. Further research using larger sample sizes and improved methodology is required in this area. Standardized measures need to be developed for use in research related to this topic.

(continued)

Evidence Table—Forearm, Wrist, and Hand (cont.)

Author/Year	Study Objectives	Level/Design/ Participants	Intervention and Outcome Measures	Results	Study Limitations	Implications for Occupational Therapy
Williams, Westmorland, Schmuck, & MacDermid, 2004 (cont.)			■ Program evaluation ■ Demographics questionnaire ■ Functional status (Modified Functional Status Scale) ■ 12 weeks of keyboard use, 24 weeks of keyboard use ■ Self-reports ■ Workplace accommodations.			

Reference: Williams, R. M., Westmorland, M. G., Schmuck, G., & MacDermid, J. C. (2004). Effectiveness of workplace rehabilitation interventions in the treatment of work-related upper extremity disorders: A systematic review. *Journal of Hand Therapy, 17,* 267–273.

Appendix E.
Evidence Table — Shoulder

Evidence Table—Shoulder

Author/Year	Study Objectives	Level/Design/ Participants	Intervention and Outcome Measures	Results	Study Limitations	Implications for Occupational Therapy
Bingol, Altan, & Yurtkuran, 2005	To assess the role of low-power gallium arsenide laser treatment in the relief of pain and the improvement of joint ROM in patients with shoulder pain	I—Randomized double-blind controlled clinical trial $N = 40$ participants with unilateral shoulder pain. Participants were assigned to an active laser treatment group or a placebo laser treatment group. Both participants and pre- and posttreatment evaluator were blinded to group placement and treatment condition. Individuals with preexisting or confounding conditions during the previous 6 months were excluded.	*Interventions:* *Active laser group:* 10 sessions of laser and exercise were performed over 2 weeks, followed by a 15-min supervised exercise program. *Placebo group:* Participants thought they were receiving laser treatment, but no laser was applied. The intervention specifics and postlaser exercise program were completed in an identical manner to the active laser group. *Outcome measures:* ■ Pain (Visual Analog Scale) ■ Palpation sensitivity ■ Goniometric measurement of the glenohumeral joint.	No significant differences were found between the groups for age, shoulder side, or pretreatment measures. Significant improvements were noted for sensitivity in the laser group and for some active and passive motions in both groups. An improvement in palpation sensitivity was noted in both groups. Comparison between the two groups showed better results in the laser group for palpation sensitivity and passive extension. No adverse reactions were noted in either group during or after the study period.	Two weeks may be inadequate to observe or measure a significant reduction in pain or a significant increase in ROM.	This study does not demonstrate that the use of low-energy laser therapy treatment for clients with unilateral shoulder pair is a significantly more efficacious preparatory modality than therapeutic exercise. The need to standardize a study design for laser treatment is necessary to clarify the role of laser as a therapeutic intervention.

Reference: Bingol, U., Altan, L., & Yurtkuran, M. (2005). Low-power laser treatment for shoulder pain. *Photomedicine and Laser Surgery, 23,* 459–464.

| Callinan et al., 2003 | To evaluate the effectiveness of hydroplasty, a hydraulic distention technique, combined with a therapy program for the treatment of idiopathic adhesive capsulitis | III—Pretest–posttest design

N = 60 participants with primary idiopathic adhesive capsulitis who had undergone hydroplasty and the subsequent therapy protocol over a 2-year period | *Interventions:*
Participants received five injections and therapy that included glenohumeral joint mobilizations and passive ROM. Participants were instructed in active and active-assistive ROM exercises to be performed 10 times each, 6 times a day. Exercises were progressed according to protocol and included dowels, pulleys, corner stretching, scapular stabilization, and postural training and education.

Outcome measures:
■ Goniometric measurement of active ROM
■ Participant self-report of pain affecting sleep
■ Total cost of surgical and therapeutic fees for hydroplasty protocol. | Significant increases were noted for all active ROM measures, both immediately posthydroplasty and at discharge. Participants with symptoms of longer duration gained significantly less ROM in internal rotation during the therapeutic phase. Those with diabetes were significantly different than those without this condition only in flexion. Pain affecting sleep was reported by 77% of participants before treatment and only 3% posttreatment. The average cost of the hydroplasty protocol was calculated to be 42% less than surgical manipulation with follow-up therapy. | There was no control group. The consistency of the therapeutic intervention and participant compliance are in question.

The study failed to analyze the differential between anterior and posterior injection sites with resultant outcomes, an additional variable that was not controlled. | The use of a hydroplasty procedure combined with therapeutic intervention is a safe and effective treatment for idiopathic adhesive capsulitis. Further prospective studies are necessary to describe specific surgical and therapeutic variables that facilitate positive outcomes. |

Reference: Callinan, N., McPherson, S., Cleaveland, S., Voss, D., Rainville, D., & Tokar, N. (2003). Effectiveness of hydroplasty and therapeutic exercise for treatment of frozen shoulder. *Journal of Hand Therapy, 16,* 219–224.

(continued)

Evidence Table—Shoulder (cont.)

Author/Year	Study Objectives	Level/Design/ Participants	Intervention and Outcome Measures	Results	Study Limitations	Implications for Occupational Therapy
Diercks & Stevens, 2004	To establish the effect of supportive therapy and supervised neglect on idiopathic frozen shoulder compared with an intensive physical therapy regimen	II—Quasi-experimental design *N* = 77 participants diagnosed with idiopathic frozen shoulder, diagnosed as more than 50% motion restriction of the glenohumeral joint in all directions for a period of >3 months Participants with preexisting or confounding conditions, including diabetes, during the past 2 years were excluded. A successive cohort served as a control group.	*Interventions:* Supportive therapy and supervised neglect group: Participants were provided an explanation of the natural course of the disease, instructed not to exercise in excess of their pain threshold, and instructed to do pendulum exercises and active exercises within this painless range and to resume all activities that were tolerated. Intensive physical therapy group: Participants were prescribed a standardized treatment protocol executed by a physical therapist of active exercises up to and beyond the pain threshold, passive stretching and manipulation of the glenohumeral joint, and home exercises aimed at stretching and maximal reaching. Whenever necessary, anti-inflammatory medications or analgesics were prescribed to participants in both groups.	At baseline, the groups did not differ significantly on pain, ROM, and functional status. During the 24-month follow-up, significant differences were found between groups at all eight measurement points. Within 2 years, 89% of participants in the supportive therapy and supervised neglect group reached a Constant score of 80 or higher, reporting no pain and almost complete glenohumeral motion; 64% of participants reached this level within 12 months. In the passive mobilization and stretching group, 63% of participants reached a Constant score of 80 or higher after 24 months, reporting no pain and almost complete glenohumeral motion.	Specific parameters of therapeutic and home exercise programs were not given for either group. A time effect cannot be ruled out secondary to study design. Finally, evaluators were not blinded to group assignment, creating a possible bias in evaluation.	Less aggressive therapeutic techniques, such as pendulum exercises, active exercises within the painless range, and tolerable functional activities, were shown to be more effective for participants with idiopathic frozen shoulder than techniques that surpass the pain threshold. Both treatment groups required at least 12 months to recover pain-free and functional glenohumeral ROM.

Outcome measures:
- Pain, ROM, and functional status (Constant score).

Reference: Diercks, R. L., & Stevens, M. (2004). Gentle thawing of the frozen shoulder: A prospective study of supervised neglect versus intensive physical therapy in seventy-seven patients with frozen shoulder syndrome followed up for two years. Journal of Shoulder and Elbow Surgery, 13, 499–502.

Author/Year	Purpose	Design/Sample	Interventions/Outcome measures	Results	Limitations	Conclusions
Ejnisman et al., 2005	To review the efficacy and safety of common interventions for tears of the rotator cuff in adults	I—Systematic review of randomized or quasi-randomized clinical trials. N = 8 trials for those with tears of the rotator cuff	Interventions: Rotator cuff tears were treated either surgically or conservatively. Outcome measures: Pain; Shoulder scores (e.g., Shoulder Pain and Disability Index); ROM; Manual muscle testing; Participant satisfaction; Reported success or failure of treatment.	None of the studies included in this review compared conservative vs. operative management of rotator cuff tears. The results provide little evidence to support or refute the efficacy of common interventions for rotator cuff tears.	Small sample size limits generalization. Methodological quality of studies included in the review was limited.	There is little evidence to support or refute conservative and/or surgical management of rotator cuff tears. Randomized studies are needed that include a uniform treatment method and core outcome measures.

Reference: Ejnisman, B., Andreoli, C. V., Soares, B. G. O., Fallopa, F., Peccin, M. S., Abdalla, R. J., et al. (2005). Interventions for tears of the rotator cuff in adults. Cochrane Database of Systematic Reviews, 1, CD002758.

Author/Year	Purpose	Design/Sample	Interventions/Outcome measures	Results	Limitations	Conclusions
Geraets et al., 2005	To assess whether graded exercise therapy is more effective than usual care after 12 weeks of treatment in restoring ability to perform daily activities irrespective of pain in patients with chronic shoulder complaints	I—Randomized clinical trial. N = 176 participants with chronic shoulder complaints lasting for >3 months. Patients with shoulder pain who had been treated in the past 3 months and those with preexisting or confounding conditions, including psychiatric diagnoses, were excluded from the study.	Interventions: Graded exercise therapy group: Treatment consisted of a behavioral program based on graded activity, time contingency, and operant conditioning and consisted of a maximum of 18 group sessions, 60 min each, over 12 weeks. Usual care group: This group received standardized treatment for shoulder	Significant differences were found between groups for the main complaint instrument and for changes in performance of activities related to participants' main complaints. Graded exercise therapy was found to have a significant and positive effect on catastrophizing. Graded exercise therapy was perceived as less effective in restoring activity of daily living	Eighteen participants withdrew from the study, and 8 were missing at posttreatment analysis.	Graded exercise therapy was shown to have a minimally greater benefit than usual care for participants with chronic shoulder pain. These results seem to be limited to participants who did not experience pain on physical exam. Further evaluation of this strategy is necessary to establish this treatment protocol as standard therapy.

(continued)

Evidence Table—Shoulder (cont.)

Author/Year	Study Objectives	Level/Design/ Participants	Intervention and Outcome Measures	Results	Study Limitations	Implications for Occupational Therapy
Geraets et al., 2005 (cont.)			complaints outlined by the Dutch College of General Practitioners that included information, recommendations, and pain-contingent medical or pharmaceutical therapy. *Outcome measures:* ▪ Daily activity measures (Main Complaints Instrument, Shoulder Disability Questionnaire [SDQ]) ▪ Perceived recovery ▪ Shoulder pain ▪ Generic health-related quality of life ▪ Catastrophizing ▪ Coping with pain ▪ Kinesiophobia ▪ Fear-Avoidance Beliefs.	(ADL) function as assessed by the SDQ for participants with a painful arc during physical examination. Overall, small beneficial effects were found for the restoration of ADL using graded exercise therapy to treat participants with chronic shoulder pain.		

Reference: Geraets, J. J. X. R., Goossens, M. E. J. B., de Groot, I. J. M., de Bruijn, C. P. C., de Bie, R. B., Dinant, G.-J., et al. (2005). Effectiveness of a graded exercise therapy program for patients with chronic shoulder complaints. *Australian Journal of Physiotherapy, 51,* 87–94.

Author/Year	Study Objectives	Level/Design/ Participants	Intervention and Outcome Measures	Results	Study Limitations	Implications for Occupational Therapy
Gibson, Growse, Korda, Wray, & MacDermid, 2004	To review the literature and determine the effectiveness of conservative management as a primary strategy in the treatment of shoulder instability. To define and identify the effectiveness of specific conservative protocols	I—Systematic review of randomized, quasi-randomized, and cohort studies and case series *N* =14 trials for those with a history of shoulder instability treated with nonoperative management	*Interventions:* Participants received nonoperative, conservative management of shoulder instability. Methods included an immobilization period of 3–4 weeks followed by a 12-week period of immobilization, stretching, strengthening, stabilization exercise, biofeedback,	Results of the review demonstrated weak yet positive support for the treatment of shoulder instability with conservative methods. One low-quality trial supported electromyography biofeedback as a beneficial adjunctive method of treatment. Conservative methods of treatment for	A critical appraisal tool has not been designed for cohort or case series designs. Foreign language articles were excluded. Common problems of individual studies included lack of randomization, control groups, blinding, and statistical analyses.	Although weak, the evidence supports a conservative program for shoulder instability that includes a 3- to 4-week immobilization period followed by 12 weeks of ROM and stability exercises. Neither ROM nor stability exercises used in isolation are recommended on the basis of this review.

		or other modalities. Relocation and splinting techniques were excluded, as well as surgical techniques not being compared to a conservative technique. *Outcome measures:* ■ Recurrence of instability, including redislocation or resubluxation ■ Functional return to work or sports activities ■ Resolution of symptoms associated with shoulder instability.		participants 30 years of age or younger provided consistently poorer outcomes than surgical management.	Electromyography biofeedback is weakly recommended as an adjunctive modality. Finally, this conservative method cannot be recommended over surgical intervention for decreasing instability recurrence.

Reference: Gibson, K., Growse, A., Korda, L., Wray, E., & MacDermid, J. C. (2004). The effectiveness of rehabilitation for nonoperative management of shoulder instability: A systematic review. *Journal of Hand Therapy, 17,* 229–242.

Grant et al., 2004	To determine the effectiveness of surgical and conservative treatments for rotator cuff pathologies To evaluate additional, lower level evidence not captured by the Cochrane systematic reviews for the treatment of rotator cuff pathologies	I—Systematic review of meta-analyses, systematic reviews, randomized controlled trials, cohort studies, and case series *N* = 4,739 (64 trials) for those who received surgical and nonsurgical interventions for rotator cuff pathologies	*Interventions:* Participants underwent surgical and nonsurgical management of rotator cuff pathology, including electrotherapy, physical therapy, exercise therapy, acupuncture therapy, shockwave therapy, laser therapy, needle aspiration, open surgical repair, mini–open surgical repair, arthroscopic surgical repair, and other surgical techniques.		Weak evidence was found to support the conservative techniques of electrotherapy, steroid injections, exercise therapy, and acupuncture. No surgical intervention was found to be more advantageous than any other.	Foreign language articles were excluded. Methodological quality of studies included in the review was mixed. Several studies had small sample sizes.	Findings from studies included in this review on rotator cuff pathology do not strongly support or refute any available intervention for this condition.

(continued)

Evidence Table—Shoulder (cont.)

Author/Year	Study Objectives	Level/Design/Participants	Intervention and Outcome Measures	Results	Study Limitations	Implications for Occupational Therapy
Grant et al., 2004 (cont.)			*Outcome measures:* ■ Pain ■ Function ■ Disability ■ Strength ■ Participant satisfaction ■ Return to work.			

Reference: Grant, H. J., Arthur, A., & Pichora, D. R. (2004). Evaluation of interventions for rotator cuff pathology: A systematic review. *Journal of Hand Therapy, 17,* 274–299.

Author/Year	Study Objectives	Level/Design/Participants	Intervention and Outcome Measures	Results	Study Limitations	Implications for Occupational Therapy
Green, Buchbinder, & Hetrick, 2003	To determine the efficacy of physical therapy interventions for disorders that result in pain, stiffness, or disability of the shoulder	I—Systematic review of randomized controlled trials *N* = 26 trials of those who experienced shoulder pain, irrespective of diagnosis	*Interventions:* Interventions included physical therapy intervention vs. placebo, no treatment, another intervention, or varied interventions. *Outcome measures:* ■ Pain ■ ROM ■ Function ■ Disability ■ Quality of life ■ Strength ■ Return to work ■ Participant perception of effect ■ Global preference ■ Physician preference ■ Adverse effects.	Weak evidence was found to support several interventions. For participants with rotator cuff disease, exercise was found to be effective in short-term recovery and long-term function, and mobilization resulted in additional benefit. When compared with placebo, laser was found to be more effective for adhesive capsulitis but not for rotator cuff disease. Also compared to placebo, ultrasound and pulsed electromagnetic field therapy were found to be beneficial for participants with calcific tendinitis. No evidence was found to support ultrasound in shoulder pain, adhesive capsulitis, or rotator cuff tendinitis; and ultrasound was not found to be beneficial	Small sample sizes of individual studies decrease generalization and increase the risk of Type II error. Interventions may not reflect those typically pursued in clinical settings.	There is weak evidence to support some interventions for pain, stiffness, and disability of the shoulder, including exercise, mobilization, laser, pulsed electromagnetic field, and ultrasound.

				compared with exercise alone. Minimal evidence exists for the use of corticosteroids over physical therapy, and there is no evidence that supports the isolated benefit of physical therapy for adhesive capsulitis.		
Reference: Green, S., Buchbinder, R., & Hetrick, S. (2003). Physiotherapy interventions for shoulder pain. *Cochrane Database of Systematic Reviews, 2,* CD004258.						
Green et al., 2006	To determine the efficacy of interventions for shoulder pain	I—Systematic review of randomized controlled trials *N* = 1,929 (31 trials) for those who experienced shoulder pain, irrespective of diagnosis	*Interventions:* Interventions included nonsteroidal anti-inflammatory drugs (NSAIDs), intra-articular and subacromial glucocorticosteroid injections, oral glucocorticosteroid treatment, physical therapy, manipulation under anesthesia, shoulder distension, and surgery. *Outcome measures:* ▪ Pain (at night, at rest, and on movement) ▪ ROM (active and/or passive: flexion, abduction, external rotation, internal rotation, and hand behind back) ▪ Function ▪ Strength ▪ Return to work or school.	This review cited a lack of uniformity in the labeling and definition of shoulder disorders, limiting the ability to pool and compare these studies. According to study authors, there is little evidence to support or refute the use of these interventions for shoulder pain. Cautious interpretation of pooled results includes increased efficacy of NSAIDs and subacromial corticosteroid injection over placebo to increase abduction for participants with rotator cuff tendinitis.	The studies in this review included subjective definitions of successful outcomes and did not report disability measurements or clinimetric properties of clinical assessments.	There is little evidence to establish the efficacy of common interventions being used to treat shoulder pain. Increased attention to sample characteristics and to standardization and objectivity of outcomes are recommended for future studies. From a clinical perspective, increased attention to objective data, including self-report outcome measures, will facilitate analysis and comparison of methods for clients with shoulder pain.
Reference: Green, S. E., Buchbinder, R., Forbes, A., & Glazier, R. (2006). Interventions for shoulder pain. *Cochrane Database of Systematic Reviews, 4,* CD001156.						

(continued)

Evidence Table—Shoulder (cont.)

Author/Year	Study Objectives	Level/Design/ Participants	Intervention and Outcome Measures	Results	Study Limitations	Implications for Occupational Therapy
Guler-Uysal & Kozano-glu, 2004	To compare early response in rehabilitation for adhesive capsulitis with attention to clinical efficacy and cost-effectiveness	I—Randomized, comparative prospective clinical trial N = 40 participants with adhesive capsulitis who met the following inclusion criteria: >2 months of pain with no major trauma, marked loss of active and passive ROM, minimum pain of 30 mm on a Visual Analog Scale during motion, normal radiographs, and absence of intervening or concomitant diagnoses	*Interventions:* A 1-week washout period was followed by blinded evaluation of pretreatment shoulder pain and ROM. In addition, serum samples and radiographs were analyzed. *Cyriax group:* Participants were seen three times a week for 1-hr sessions of deep friction massage and manipulation performed by the same therapist. *Physical therapy group:* Participants were seen five times a week for 1-hr sessions of a 20 min superficial heat (hot pack) treatment followed by 20 min of short-wave diathermy in a supine position. Both groups performed active stretching and pendulum exercises after each session, and both groups had a standardized home exercise program. NSAIDs and analgesics were not permitted during the study.	At the end of the 2nd week, 19 of 20 participants in the Cyriax group achieved the expected outcome, compared with 13 of 20 in the physical therapy group, a significant difference. Glenohumeral flexion, internal and external rotation, and decreased pain were significantly improved in the Cyriax group. In addition, the Cyriax group had a significantly lower number of treatment sessions over the 2-week period.	Specific information regarding home exercise programs in terms of repetition and duration were not discussed. Participant compliance with exercises was not measured or discussed. Long-term follow-up data were not reported.	The Cyriax method of rehabilitation, including deep friction massage and joint manipulation, was shown to produce significantly greater changes in glenohumeral flexion, rotations, and pain in a significantly decreased amount of treatment time compared with therapy using superficial and deep heat treatments. The Cyriax method is suggested as a beneficial preparatory activity to purposeful and occupation-based activities. Larger sample sizes and long-term follow-up are recommended for future research.

Outcome measures:

- Recovery rate (number of participants who achieved 80% of normal ROM at the end of the 2nd week of the study).

Reference: Guler-Uysal, F., & Kozanoglu, E. (2004). Comparison of the early response of two methods of rehabilitation in adhesive capsulitis. *Swiss Medical Weekly, 134,* 353–358.

Haldorsen et al., 2002	To determine effective treatments, investigate the use of a screening tool, and identify benefits to society of treatment for employees with musculoskeletal pain on long-term sick leave	I—Randomized controlled trial *N* = 654 participants on long-term sick leave from work Participants were screened into three levels of prognosis (good, medium, poor) and randomly assigned to three different treatments (ordinary, light multidisciplinary, and extensive multidisciplinary).	*Interventions:* *Ordinary treatment group:* Participants were referred back to their general practitioner, who gave medication, advice, and further referrals to physiotherapists or chiropractors. *Light multidisciplinary group:* Participants received a 1-hr lecture and were encouraged to increase their activity level even if pain was present. Each participant received an individualized exercise program based on physical tests. *Extensive multidisciplinary treatment:* Treatment program lasted 4 weeks and included 6-hr sessions 5 days a week that incorporated cognitive–behavioral treatment, education sessions, and an individualized exercise program.	This study found that the use of a screening instrument could identify the prognosis of return to work in participants with musculoskeletal pain. Both the light and extensive multidisciplinary treatments increased the possibility of return to work compared with the ordinary treatment, independent of screening category. For those who had a good prognosis, ordinary treatment was found to be sufficient. Those with a medium prognosis benefited equally from multidisciplinary treatments, and those with poor prognoses were found to return to work at a significantly higher rate when receiving extensive multidisciplinary treatment. Nine in 10 participants had been out of work for at least 8 weeks. Return to work was the only outcome measurement used in this study; quality of life was not taken into account.	The use of a screening tool is beneficial, especially for clients with a poor prognosis. A screening tool is also beneficial to health professionals in that it addresses psychological and motivational aspects resulting in better treatment effects. The consideration of prognosis as a means to guide the course of intervention has been demonstrated to have a significant impact on return to work. This information could be used to establish the optimal number of visits and skill mix necessary for goal-directed outcomes.

(continued)

Evidence Table—Shoulder (cont.)

Author/Year	Study Objectives	Level/Design/Participants	Intervention and Outcome Measures	Results	Study Limitations	Implications for Occupational Therapy
Haldorsen et al., 2002 (cont.)			At the end of the program, participants developed their own rehabilitation plan and were followed up for 1 year. *Outcome measures:* ■ Return to work ■ Follow-up data collected from the social insurance register regarding duration, amount of sickness benefits, rehabilitation benefits, and disability pension.			
Handoll & Almaiyah, 2004	To compare surgical versus nonsurgical treatment for acute anterior dislocation of the shoulder	I—Systematic review of randomized or quasi-randomized controlled trials *N* = 5 trials of those who had undergone surgical or conservative interventions for acute anterior dislocation of the shoulder	*Interventions:* Surgical interventions, both open and minimally invasive, were compared with nonsurgical interventions for acute anterior shoulder dislocation. *Primary outcome measures:* ■ Return to preinjury level of activity (sports or work) ■ Reinjury or recurrence ■ Persistent pain ■ Subjective instability ■ Results from validated self-report outcome measures.	Instability following treatment was significantly less frequent in the surgical group, and half of the participants who received nonsurgical treatment opted for subsequent surgery. The majority of self-report measures revealed significantly better outcomes for participants treated surgically. Types of surgery differed across trials, as did length of immobilization and rehabilitation.	Small sample sizes limit generalization. Return to activity was reported differently across trials, and outcomes varied within trials.	There is limited evidence to support primary surgery for young men who have sustained their first acute traumatic shoulder dislocation and who are engaged in highly demanding physical activities. No evidence currently supports the method of surgery or the use of primary surgery for other client groups.

Reference: Haldorsen, E. M., Grasdal, A. L., Skouen, J. S., Risa, A. E., Skronholm, K., & Ursin, H. (2002). Is there a right treatment for a particular patient group? Comparison of ordinary treatment, light multidisciplinary treatment, and extensive multidisciplinary treatment for long-term sick-listed employees with musculoskeletal pain. *Pain, 95,* 49–63.

Secondary outcome measures:
- Objective instability
- Stiffness
- ROM
- Muscle strength
- Complications
- Satisfaction.

Reference:. Handoll, H. H. G., & Almaiyah, M. A. (2004). Surgical versus nonsurgical treatment for acute anterior shoulder dislocation. *Cochrane Database of Systematic Reviews, 1,* CD004325.

| Handoll, Gibson, & Madhok, 2003 | To gather and assess the evidence for various methods of treating proximal humeral fractures | I—Systematic review of randomized and quasi-randomized controlled trials

N = 578 participants (12 trials) with proximal humeral fractures | *Interventions:*
Conservative and surgical interventions were used to treat or rehabilitate proximal humeral fractures, including immobilization, closed reduction and K-wire stabilization, external fixation, open reduction and plating, open reduction and wiring, antegrade or retrograde intramedullary nailing, hemiarthroplasty, and total shoulder replacement.

Outcome measures:
• Anatomical reduction as demonstrated by radiological deformity of the proximal humeral angle
• Clinical outcomes including strength, ROM, pain, satisfaction, and complications
• Functional outcomes including health-related quality of life | This review provided limited evidence for type of bandage as indicative of fracture healing and functional outcomes, some evidence that immediate therapy resulted in less pain and both faster and better recovery for participants with nondisplaced two-part fractures, some evidence that mobilization at 1 week alleviated short-term pain, and some evidence that participants could achieve a satisfactory outcome without supervised therapy.

Operative treatment resulted in improved fracture alignment, better function, and less pain with hemiarthroplasty compared with conservative treatment. There was very limited evidence that early mobilization following surgery makes a difference in outcomes. | Small sample sizes limit generalization. | There is limited evidence to support decision making for the management of proximal humeral fractures. Occupational therapists may appropriately pursue early therapeutic intervention without immobilization for specific, nondisplaced fractures. The long-term benefits of surgical intervention are unclear. |

(continued)

Evidence Table—Shoulder (cont.)

Author/Year	Study Objectives	Level/Design/ Participants	Intervention and Outcome Measures	Results	Study Limitations	Implications for Occupational Therapy
Handoll, Gibson, & Madhok, 2003 *(cont.)*			▪ Economic outcomes including attendance at outpatient appointments.			

Reference: Handoll, H. H. G., Gibson, J. N. A., & Madhok, R. (2003). Interventions for treating proximal humerus fractures in adults. *Cochrane Database of Systematic Reviews, 4,* CD000434.

Handoll et al., 2006	To compare nonsurgical intervention methods following closed reduction of traumatic anterior dislocation of the shoulder	I—Systematic review of randomized and quasi-randomized controlled trials *N* = 40 participants (1 trial) who had undergone closed reduction of traumatic anterior dislocation of the shoulder	*Interventions:* Participants received postoperative management that included differing methods, positions, durations, and extent of immobilization, as well as differing rehabilitation interventions, including education, ROM, and exercise. *Primary outcome measures:* ▪ Return to preinjury level of activity (sports or work) ▪ Reinjury or recurrence ▪ Persistent pain ▪ Subjective instability ▪ Results from validated self-report outcome measures. *Secondary outcome measures:* ▪ Objective instability ▪ ROM ▪ Muscle strength ▪ Complications ▪ Satisfaction ▪ Adherence to allocated treatment.	There were no significant differences among participants in functional outcomes, including redislocation or instability.	Small sample size limits its generalization. Only one study was included in the review. Removal of the immobilization device by participants may have affected results.	This study does not provide sufficient evidence to inform conservative management following closed reduction of traumatic anterior dislocation of the shoulder.

Reference: Handoll, H. H. G., Hanchard, N. C. A., Goodchild, L., & Feary, J. (2006). Conservative management following closed reduction of traumatic anterior dislocation of the shoulder. *Cochrane Database of Systematic Reviews, 1,* CD004962.

| Jurgel et al., 2005 | To examine shoulder active ROM, shoulder muscle maximal isometric force, and endurance in patients with frozen shoulder in both the involved and uninvolved extremity before and after treatment | III—Case control design including a group with frozen shoulder and a comparison group with asymptomatic shoulders

N = 10 participants with frozen shoulder in the treatment group and 10 control group participants who were similar in age and gender to the treatment group | *Interventions:*
Those in the frozen shoulder group received a 4-week rehabilitation program performed by the same physiotherapist consisting of 10 individualized exercise procedures for 30 min per day, 5–10 massage procedures 20 min per day, and 5–10 electrical therapy procedures 5–10 min per day.

Outcome measures:
■ Shoulder active ROM
■ Shoulder muscle isometric strength and endurance. | After rehabilitation, participants with frozen shoulder were noted to have increased shoulder flexion, extension, and abduction-active ROM of the involved extremity. However, these measurements remained significantly lower than in the uninvolved extremity and the control group. Maximal force of the external and internal rotators of the participants with frozen shoulder was increased but remained significantly lower than in the uninvolved extremity. Maximal force of shoulder external rotators on the involved extremity increased but remained significantly lower than in the control group. No significant differences in muscle endurance in the frozen shoulder group were observed compared with the uninvolved extremity or the control group. | A 4-week rehabilitation program may not be long enough to observe significant increases in shoulder function. The study had a relatively small sample size and may not be generalized to all clients with frozen shoulder. | A rehabilitation program can improve active ROM and muscle strength of the shoulder in clients with frozen shoulder. To promote more significant changes, exercise therapy of higher intensity and duration along with other treatments should be conducted. Clients should also do exercises at home. |

Reference: Jurgel, J., Rannama, L., Gapeyeva, H., Ereline, J., Kolts, I., & Paasuke, M. (2005). Shoulder function in patients with frozen shoulder before and after 4-week rehabilitation. *Medicina (Kaunas), 41,* 30–38.

(continued)

Evidence Table—Shoulder (cont.)

Author/Year	Study Objectives	Level/Design/Participants	Intervention and Outcome Measures	Results	Study Limitations	Implications for Occupational Therapy
Karjalainen et al., 2003	To determine the effectiveness of multidisciplinary biopsychosocial rehabilitation for adults with neck and shoulder pain	I—Systematic review of randomized and non-randomized controlled trials N = 2 trials for those with neck and shoulder pain	*Interventions:* Participants received multidisciplinary inpatient or outpatient programs that included consultation with a physician as well as a psychological, social, or vocational intervention or some combination. *Outcome measures:* ■ Pain intensity ■ Global status ■ Disorder-specific functional status ■ Generic functional status and quality of life ■ Ability to work ■ Health care consumption and costs ■ Satisfaction with treatments.	Neither study provided sufficient evidence to support multidisciplinary biopsychosocial rehabilitation programs as beneficial for working-age adults with neck and shoulder pain.	Small sample sizes limit generalization. Both studies were of low quality.	There is little scientific evidence to support multidisciplinary biopsychosocial rehabilitation programs as beneficial for adults with neck and shoulder pain. As this is a common intervention approach, high-quality trials in this area are urgently needed.

Reference: Karjalainen, K., Malmivaara, A., van Tulder, M., Roine, R., Jauhiainen, M., Hurri, H., et al. (2003). Multidisciplinary biopsychosocial rehabilitation for neck and shoulder pain in working age adults. *Cochrane Database of Systematic Reviews, 3,* CD002194.

Author/Year	Study Objectives	Level/Design/Participants	Intervention and Outcome Measures	Results	Study Limitations	Implications for Occupational Therapy
Ludewig & Borstad, 2003	To implement and evaluate a therapeutic exercise program intended to modify shoulder elevation and muscle activity abnormalities believed to be related to shoulder impingement	I—Randomized controlled trial N = 103 construction workers with occupational exposure to overhead work for longer than 1 year, current shoulder pain localized to the glenohumeral joint, pain in the C5–6 dermatome present with at least two positive shoulder impingement tests,	*Interventions:* Participants in the intervention group were given a home exercise program consisting of stretches, muscle relaxation exercises, and progressive resistance strengthening exercises and were asked to keep a compliance log. Both the intervention and control groups returned at 10 weeks	The intervention group showed significant improvements in SRQ scores and in satisfaction. Both symptomatic and asymptomatic control groups showed no change in functional status or pain. At the end of the study, work-related pain and disability scores of the intervention group were significantly	Convenience sample of male construction workers limits generalization to female construction workers or other workers who complete overhead tasks. The study is specific to shoulder impingement and rotator cuff tendinitis; further research is needed to determine the effects of the home exercise pro-	This study supports the use of a shoulder home exercise program to improve shoulder function and reduction in symptoms for construction workers who have routine exposure to overhead work. Further research should be done to test the home exercise program on other populations and to

(continued)

Objective	Design / Participants	Intervention & Outcome Measures	Results	Limitations / Conclusions
investigate the effects of a home exercise program on clients following rotator cuff surgeries and other shoulder injuries. … gram in treatment of nonspecific shoulder pain.	and reproduced pain during two of the three clinical tests. There were $n = 34$ in the intervention group, $n = 33$ in a no treatment control group, and these groups were the result of randomization. There were an additional $n = 25$ asymptomatic volunteers in the second control group. Asymptomatic participants formed one control group. Participants were excluded who had a history of rotator cuff surgery, a history of glenohumeral dislocation or other traumatic injury to the shoulder, only periscapular or cervical pain during elevation, or shoulder symptoms that were reproduced by a cervical assessment.	for a follow-up visit. At this point the control groups were instructed in the exercise program. *Outcome measures:* ■ Shoulder pain, disability, and satisfaction (Shoulder Rating Questionnaire [SRQ] and additional questions)	reduced compared with those of the symptomatic control group; however, they remained significantly greater than those of the a symptomatic group.	

Reference: Ludewig, P. M., & Borstad, J. D. (2003). Effects of a home exercise programme on shoulder pain and functional status in construction workers. *Occupational and Environmental Medicine, 60,* 841–849.

| Lundblad, Elert, & Gerdle, 1999 | To compare physical therapy with Feldenkrais interventions in the reduction of complaints of the neck and shoulder | I—Randomized controlled trial. $N = 97$ female industrial trial workers with neck and shoulder pain. Participants were excluded who had long-term illness, previous attempts at intensive rehabilitation, difficulty with the Swedish | *Interventions:* The physical therapy group met 2 times a week for 50 min in small groups of 5–8 and focused on education, stabilizing exercises for the low back and pelvis, isolated and relaxed shoulder movements to control the muscles, awareness of body postures, | A significantly higher proportion of participants in the Feldenkrais group than in the control group showed improvements in the neck shoulder index. The Feldenkrais group also showed a significant decrease in neck and shoulder complaints, whereas the complaints from the other two groups were | The study had a high number of dropouts. The study included only female industrial workers, limiting generalization. The Feldenkrais method has commonalities with relaxation and biofeedback techniques, which have both been shown to decrease pain. Feldenkrais therapy was demonstrated in this study to be a holistic preparatory intervention that facilitates return to work. Further research is needed |

Evidence Table—Shoulder (cont.)

Author/Year	Study Objectives	Level/Design/ Participants	Intervention and Outcome Measures	Results	Study Limitations	Implications for Occupational Therapy
Lundblad, Elert, & Gerdle, 1999 (cont.)		language, pregnancy, coronary disease, rheumatoid arthritis, rotator cuff tendinitis, and plans to leave the job during the study.	work-related lift and movement techniques, and an exercise program (strengthening, coordination, endurance, flexibility, rhythm). The Feldenkrais group received individual treatment 4 times and group treatment 12 times. Participants received audiocassettes providing instruction in exercises to increase awareness of sensory afferents; investigate unconscious tension, posture, and movement patterns; break stereotyped movement patterns; and enable self-care for pain in the neck, shoulders, and back. Intervention lasted 50 min per week. The control group received no intervention. *Outcome measures:* ▪ Neck shoulder index ▪ Pain ▪ Measures of disability, including sick leave.	unchanged. Pain intensity decreased the most in the Feldenkrais group. Although there was no difference between groups in length of sick leave from work, there was a statistically significant decrease in disability for the Feldenkrais group with respect to leisure participation.		to justify Feldenkrais interventions for people with neck or shoulder complaints.

Reference: Lundblad, I., Elert, J., & Gerdle, B. (1999). Randomized controlled trial of physiotherapy and Feldenkrais interventions in female workers with neck-shoulder complaints. *Journal of Occupational Rehabilitation, 9*, 179–194.

Author/Year	Study Objectives	Level/Design/Participants	Intervention and Outcome Measures	Results	Study Limitations	Implications for Occupational Therapy
Michener, Walsworth, & Burnet, 2004	To examine the efficacy of nonsurgical and nonpharmacological rehabilitation of subacromial impingement syndrome	I—Systematic review of randomized clinical trials and clinical trials N = 12 trials for those with subacromial impingement syndrome	*Interventions:* Participants engaged in exercise, joint mobilization, laser, ultrasound, and acupuncture performed in combination or in isolation. *Outcome measures:* - Pain - Functional loss or disability.	This review revealed limited evidence to support exercise for strengthening of the rotator cuff and scapular musculature and stretching of the surrounding soft tissues. Joint mobilizations were found to increase effectiveness of this type of exercise. In addition, laser appears to be beneficial when used in isolation, the use of ultrasound for this population was not supported, and acupuncture yielded equivocal results.	Small sample sizes limit generalization. Foreign language articles were excluded.	There is limited evidence to support exercise and joint mobilizations for clients with subacromial impingement syndrome.

Reference: Michener, L. A., Walsworth, M. K., & Burnet, E. N. (2004). Effectiveness of rehabilitation for patients with subacromial impingement syndrome: A systematic review. *Journal of Hand Therapy, 17,* 152–164.

Author/Year	Study Objectives	Level/Design/Participants	Intervention and Outcome Measures	Results	Study Limitations	Implications for Occupational Therapy
Novak, Collins, & Mackinnon, 1995	To evaluate long-term subjective outcomes following conservative management of patients with thoracic outlet syndrome (TOS) using posture modification and a specific physical therapy program	III—Cross-sectional survey N = 42 participants who had a clinical diagnosis of TOS Participants were divided into three groups: symptomatic intervention, symptomatic control, and asymptomatic control.	*Interventions:* During the initial visit, all participants were educated on postures and positions that could contribute to TOS symptoms or brachial plexus compression. Then the participants were given an exercise program consisting of graduated stretching and strengthening. *Outcome measures:* - Past symptoms - Present symptoms - Participant opinion regarding the therapy program - Medication - Employment status - Demographic data.	Twenty-five participants reported that their present symptoms were better than before treatment, 10 reported no change, and 7 had worse pain. Fifteen of the 16 participants who had no change with previous therapy reported improvement of neck and shoulder symptoms. In total, 38 participants experienced relief of neck and shoulder pain, and 27 experienced relief of hand and arm symptoms. Participants who were overweight or had carpal tunnel syndrome were significantly less likely to report full or almost complete pain relief.	This study had no actual control group, making it hard to determine the true effectiveness of the exercise program. The small sample size limits its generalization.	This study supports the effectiveness of conservative management in treating TOS. A home exercise program was found to reduce pain in the proximal regions of the body. Further studies should be pursued to determine the effects of factors such as obesity, breast hypertrophy, and demographic variables on outcomes of TOS.

(continued)

Evidence Table—Shoulder (cont.)

Author/Year	Study Objectives	Level/Design/ Participants	Intervention and Outcome Measures	Results	Study Limitations	Implications for Occupational Therapy

Reference: Novak, C. B., Collins, E. D., & Mackinnon, S. E. (1995). Outcome following conservative management of thoracic outlet syndrome. *Journal of Hand Surgery, 20A,* 542–548.

| Piotte et al., 2004 | To evaluate the combined effectiveness of repeated distention arthrographies (DA) with a home exercise program for patients with adhesive capsulitis of the shoulder | III—Repeated measures design

N = 15 participants with primary idiopathic adhesive capsulitis, pain for >3 months, and >30% loss of range of two motions of the shoulder compared with the contralateral side

All participants reported previous treatment, and 2 reported previous issues with the contralateral shoulder. | *Interventions:*
Participants were taught a home exercise program including either active or active assisted ROM depending on pain and evaluative measurements. One of two radiologists then performed the first DA in a standardized fashion using an anterior approach with participants supine. Two additional evaluations followed by DAs were performed at 3-week intervals. With each evaluation, home exercise programs were changed according to changes in ROM. A final evaluation was performed 3 weeks after the final DA. Participants recorded the use of ice and acetaminophen for pain control at home.

Outcome measures:
■ Pain and shoulder history (Shoulder Pain and Disability Index)
■ Active and passive ROM in supine
■ Pain-free strength (dynamometer). | A significant improvement was found in all measures at the conclusion of intervention, with the greatest effects occurring after the first DA, less marked yet significant effects occurring after the second DA, and minimal effects occurring after the third DA. Following intervention, significant differences in ROM were noted compared with the contralateral side. | This study used a repeated measures design with no controls, so it is impossible to differentiate the effectiveness of DA and home exercise programs. Dissociation of effects of subsequent DAs from previous ones is impossible. A small sample size that was primarily female limits generalization to the greater population. | Occupational therapists can contribute to protocols such as these that combine DA and preparatory activities.

Further prospective studies are necessary to delineate specific surgical and therapeutic variables that facilitate positive outcomes. |

Reference: Piotte, F., Gravel, D., Moffet, H., Fliszar, E., Roy, A., Nadeau, S., et al. (2004). Effects of repeated distension arthrographies combined with a home exercise program among adults with idiopathic adhesive capsulitis of the shoulder. *American Journal of Physical Medicine and Rehabilitation, 83,* 537–546.

Randlov et al., 1998	To compare the effectiveness of two types of training on chronic neck and shoulder pain	I—Randomized controlled trial *N* = 77 women ages 18–65 with chronic neck or shoulder pain for >6 months. Participants were randomly assigned to receive an intensive training program or a lighter training program.	*Interventions:* *Intensive training group:* Participants began with bicycling and stretching exercises of relevant muscle groups (neck and shoulder). The shoulder exercises were carried out with increasing resistance. *Lighter training group:* Each session began with applying hot packs followed by stationary bicycling and stretching of relevant muscle groups. *Outcome measures:* ■ Pain (11-point box scales) ■ ADL (disability scale) ■ Maximal voluntary isometric contraction of the flexors and extensors of the cervical spine (strain gauge equipment).	There were significant improvements in ADL scores within both groups but no significant difference in improvement between groups. Although pain scores for the intensive training group were significantly lower at 12-month follow-up, no significant differences were found between the two groups. The overall success rate was 50% at the conclusion of treatment and 60% at the 12-month follow-up.	The two interventions were similar, which may have resulted in the lack of significant differences between groups. The study did not include a control group, which makes it difficult to determine the effectiveness of each treatment. The study included only women, limiting generalizability.	The use of both intensive training and lighter training was shown to be beneficial in improving function for clients with chronic neck and shoulder pain.

Reference: Randlov, A., Ostergaard, M., Manniche, C., Kryger, P., Jordan, A., Heegard, S., et al. (1998). Intensive dynamic training for females with chronic neck/shoulder pain: A randomized controlled trial. *Clinical Rehabilitation, 12,* 200–210.

(continued)

Evidence Table—Shoulder (cont.)

Author/Year	Study Objectives	Level/Design/ Participants	Intervention and Outcome Measures	Results	Study Limitations	Implications for Occupational Therapy
Ryans et al., 2005	To examine the effectiveness of intra-articular steroid treatment and physiotherapy alone and in combination for patients with adhesive capsulitis	I—Randomized controlled trial *N* = 80 participants with painful shoulder lasting 4 weeks to 18 months recruited from local general practices Participants were assigned to an injection and physiotherapy group (Group A), an injection and no physiotherapy group (Group B), a placebo injection and physiotherapy group (Group C), and a placebo injection and no physiotherapy group (Group D). Both participants and investigator were blinded to the nature of the injection.	*Interventions:* Groups A and B were administered injections by a single experienced clinician. Half of the solution was injected in the anterior shoulder and the other half in the lateral subacromial space. Physiotherapy took place in eight sessions over a 4-week period and included standardized treatment. *Outcome measures:* ■ Anxiety and depression (SF-36) ■ Active and passive ROM ■ Shoulder disability ■ Pain at rest ■ Self-assessment of global function.	At 6 weeks, significant improvement in shoulder disability questionnaire scores and participant global assessment was noted for participants who had received the injection. The physiotherapy group experienced significant improvement of passive external rotation. No significant improvements were found for pain at rest in any of the groups. At 16 weeks, no significant differences were found between interventions in any outcome measures. Eight participants were dissatisfied with their outcome (5 from Group D and 3 from Group C) and were offered further treatment.	Injections were given under radiological guidance, limiting generalization to clinical practice. Attrition may have affected the findings after 16 weeks.	Improvements were seen with injection and physiotherapy, but no interaction between the two was found. This shows that positive effects of the treatments may be seen in different aspects of dysfunction. This study used injections in the anterior and lateral portions of the shoulder, but other studies have used different methods. Further research is needed to determine the most effective approach to injection.

Reference: Ryans, I., Montgomery, A., Galway, R., Kernohan, W. G., & McKane, R. (2005). A randomized controlled trial of intra-articular triamcinolone and/or physiotherapy in shoulder capsulitis. *Rheumatology, 44,* 529–535.

| Sjogren et al., 2005 | To test the effects of a workplace intervention on headaches, neck and shoulder symptoms, and upper extremity strength in office workers | II—Cluster randomized controlled trial

N = 53 office workers with headache, shoulder, or neck pain during the previous 12 months that restricted daily activities; these workers performed physically light work. | *Interventions:*
The exercise–resistence group did physical exercise and light resistance training guided by a physical therapist in three sessions at 5-week intervals. | This study found that physical exercise resulted in a slight, yet significant, decrease in headache and neck symptoms as well as an increase in extension strength. No effects on shoulder symptoms or flexion strength were noted. | Sample size and population drawn from limits its generalization to the greater population of clients who complain of head, neck, and shoulder pain. | There is limited evidence that daily, light resistance training guided by a therapist can decrease head and neck symptoms and increase shoulder extension strength for clients who perform physically light work. |

	Participants were allocated to two treatment sequence groups: exercise–resistance intervention and no physical exercise intervention.	*Outcome measures:* ■ Perceived exertion (Borg Rating of Perceived Exertion) ■ Pain.		

Reference: Sjogren, T., Nissinen, K. J., Jarvenpaa, S. K., Ojanen, M. T., Vanharanta, H., & Malkia, E. A. (2005). Effects of a workplace physical exercise intervention on the intensity of headache and neck and shoulder symptoms and upper extremity muscular strength of office workers: A cluster randomized controlled cross-over trial. *Pain, 116,* 119–128.

Vermeulen, Rozing, Obermann, le Cessie, & Vliet Vleland, 2006	To compare the effectiveness of high-grade mobilization techniques for patients with adhesive capsulitis of the shoulder	I—Randomized controlled study *N* = 100 participants with unilateral adhesive capsulitis for >3 months and >50% decrease in passive ROM compared with the contralateral side Participants were randomly assigned to the high-grade mobilization technique (HGMT) group or the low-grade mobilization technique (LGMT) group.	*Interventions:* Both groups were treated two times a week for 30 min for a maximum of 12 weeks. At the conclusion of each treatment, passive proprioceptive neuromuscular facilitation patterns and active pendulum exercises were completed. Use of pain medication during the treatment phase was monitored for both groups. HGMT is intensive passive mobilization in end-range positions of the glenohumeral joint while in LGMT, participants were treated with passive mobilization within the pain-free zone. *Outcome measures:* ■ Active and passive ROM ■ Shoulder Rating Questionnaire (SRQ) ■ Shoulder Disabilities Questionnaire (SDQ) ■ Pain (Visual Analog Scale) ■ SF–36.	Both groups improved significantly over 12 months. Significant improvements in passive abduction and active and passive external rotation were found for the HGMT group. The HGMT group was also found to have a significant trend difference in passive external rotation and SRQ and SDQ scores over 12 months compared with the LGMT group.	Absence of a control group limits the ability to analyze the effectiveness of LGMT compared with placebo or no treatment. Small sample size limits ability to detect small differences between treatment groups. Participants generally had a long duration of shoulder complaints, and therefore this study cannot be generalized to all clients with adhesive capsulitis. There is limited evidence to support the efficacy of high-grade mobilization techniques compared with low-grade mobilization techniques for the improvement of shoulder mobility and reduction of self-reported disability in clients with phase II adhesive capsulitis.

(continued)

Author/Year	Study Objectives	Level/Design/ Participants	Intervention and Outcome Measures	Results	Study Limitations	Implications for Occupational Therapy

Reference: Vermeulen, H. M., Rozing, P. M., Obermann, W. R., le Cessie, S., & Vliet Vleland, T. P. M. (2006). Comparison of high-grade and low-grade mobilization techniques in the management of adhesive capsulitis of the shoulder: Randomized controlled trial. *Physical Therapy, 86,* 355–368.

Author/Year	Study Objectives	Level/Design/ Participants	Intervention and Outcome Measures	Results	Study Limitations	Implications for Occupational Therapy
Waling, Sundelin, Ahlgren, & Jarvholm, 2000	To evaluate the effectiveness of strength, endurance, and coordination programs on neck and shoulder pain in women with work-related trapezius myalgia	I—Randomized controlled trial *N* = 126 participants who were employed and reported at least 1 year of neck or shoulder problems Participants were excluded if they had been on sick leave for >1 month in the year before the study. Participants were randomized into three exercise groups and one nonexercise (control) group.	*Interventions:* Participants in the three exercise groups received training in strength (concentric resistance exercise), endurance (ergometer, abdominal and back exercises), or coordination (body awareness therapy). The control group participated in a 12-week stress management program. *Outcome measures:* ■ Pain at present, pain at worst (Visual Analog Scale) ■ Pain trigger points (Somedic pressure algometer) ■ Pain drawings ■ Subjective evaluation of training effects on symptoms (5 graded categorical scale).	Pain at worst decreased significantly in the strength and endurance groups. Pressure sensitivity decreased significantly in four trigger points in the exercise groups. Comparison of exercise groups with the control group showed significant reductions in pain at present and at worst in the exercise groups. All exercise groups showed similar decreases in pain.	Small sample size limits ability to detect minor changes in pain. Voluntary recruitment technique limits applicability to all female workers. The control group constituted a fourth intervention group, rather than a no treatment group; the control group used, however, helps eliminate the attention bias that may have occurred if a no treatment control group was used.	There is limited evidence to support the efficacy of exercise programs to reduce pain caused by work-related trapezius myalgia.

Reference: Waling, K., Sundelin, G., Ahlgren, C., & Jarvholm, B. (2000). Perceived pain before and after three exercise programs—A controlled clinical trial of women with work-related trapezius myalgia. *Pain, 85,* 201–207.

Appendix F. Utilization Guidelines and Occupational Therapy

Utilization management of therapy services is a major concern for workers' compensation payers, providers, and clients. Individual state workers' compensation boards and commercial entities such as the *Official Disability Guidelines Treatment* (Work Loss Data Institute; Denniston, 2008), the *Medical Disability Advisor* (Reed Group; Reed, 2005), and the *Occupational Medicine Practice Guidelines* (American College of Occupational and Environmental Medicine; Glass, 2004) have developed several medical guidelines. However, the role of rehabilitation therapies generally, and occupational therapy specifically, has historically received inadequate attention with regard to return-to-work analysis. Some medical guidelines draw on extensive databases and attempt to combine treatment guidelines with disability duration benchmarks specifically for the workers' compensation population. Although this is a positive step toward answering the difficult question of how much lost time can be expected before a person returns to work, "potential benefits will be negated if any party resents the guidelines or questions the validity of the source" (Stutzman, 2001, p. 37).

In most existing guidelines, references to occupational therapy are either missing or aggregated into sections that refer to "physical therapy" as a generic treatment. Regardless of which overall guidelines workers' compensation payers incorporate into their claims management systems, in addition to having norms, guidelines should identify what makes a difference in return to work for a specific condition (Prezzia & Denniston, 2001). Using normative numbers without considering the additional factors affecting the client and the return-to-work environment will not ensure a good outcome for the client, employer, provider, or workers'

compensation insurer (Stutzman, 2001). This appendix provides an overview of often-overlooked factors that could significantly affect successful return to work.

AOTA Survey of Occupational Therapy Practitioners

In addition to the evidence-based literature review presented in this guideline, AOTA conducted online surveys of occupational therapists whose areas of practice included postacute services to individuals with work-related injuries or illnesses of the upper extremity and low back under workers' compensation payment systems. This information is intended to supplement the evidence-based material found in this and other guidelines and to provide additional insight into relationships among occupational therapy utilization, clients' functional needs, and workers' compensation system requirements. Occupational therapists treat individuals with many of the same diagnoses under other insurance plans and provide services in other programs where work is a goal, such as employer on-site ergonomics training, vocational rehabilitation, and wellness or prevention programs. However, our questionnaire was limited solely to treatment of clients receiving postacute services under workers' compensation.

We requested expert opinion on the "typical" frequency and duration for a continuous episode of care for clients, classified within a specific group of diagnoses, whose ultimate goal is to return to work either in a previous employment category or an alternate job choice. We defined *typical* for the purpose of this survey as the frequency and duration range that would be appropriate for the majority of patients with the specified diagnoses. More importantly, we requested information on the nature of clinical, patient-specific, and environmental factors that would likely result in increases or decreases in utilization.

We reviewed all of the combination visit and duration data for the upper extremity and low back diagnoses to determine the extent to which utilization for a typical client could be defined within a diagnostic group. Table F1 lists the findings regarding the types of conditions for which a typical client would receive greater or less than 4 weeks of occupational therapy, based solely on the diagnosis (numbers in parentheses are *ICD-9-CM* codes; Ameican Medical Association, 2008). A great deal of variation in numbers of visits and weeks of therapy was reported across diagnoses, which may be attributed to a wide range of influences such as policy differences in workers' compensation systems across the country, the protocols followed by individual physicians and therapists, and other factors that affect the intensity of therapy.

Factors That Affect Frequency and Duration of Occupational Therapy Services

Studies that have looked at utilization suggest that the medical diagnosis (i.e., *ICD-9-CM* code) may not be a good determinant of therapy outcomes. As stated in a report by the National Committee on Vital and Health Statistics (2002),

> Most diagnoses alone convey little about their effects on people's daily activities or the impact of people's social or physical environments. Diagnosis does not reveal or predict function—and function has an enormous effect on utilization rates and is a good indicator of quality of care, among other things. (p. 7)

From a small group of occupational therapists across the country treating workers' compensation clients with upper extremity and low back conditions, we requested lists of "person factors" (e.g., comorbidities, internal motivation) and "service delivery factors" (e.g., environmental or system factors, other factors external to the person) that most affect utilization of occupational therapy services; the factors they identified are listed in Table F2. We requested that all survey respondents rate each factor according to the extent to which it has an effect on occupational therapy utilization using a five-point scale ranging from *always* to *none*. To analyze the results, we combined the ratings into two classifications (*often/always* and *none/very limited/sometimes*). We also requested that respondents provide open-ended comments regarding variances in treatment utilization.

The analysis and comments the therapists provided echoed some of the improved outcome attributions

Table F1. Duration of Occupational Therapy, Based Solely on Diagnosis

Area	Condition
More than 60% of respondents reported that their typical client received 1–4 weeks of occupational therapy for the following conditions:	
Upper extremity	Mononeuritis of upper limb and mononeuritis multiplex (354)

	Superficial injury of
	  Shoulder and upper arm (912)
	  Hand(s) except finger(s) alone (914)
	  Finger(s) (915)

	Contusion of upper limb
	  Shoulder and upper arm (923.0)
	  Elbow and forearm (923.1)
	  Wrist and hand(s) (923.2)
	  Finger(s) (923.3)

Table F1. Duration of Occupational Therapy, Based Solely on Diagnosis *(cont.)*

Area	Condition

More than 80% of respondents reported that their typical client received more than 4 weeks or more than 4 visits per week of occupational therapy for the following conditions:

Area	Condition

Upper extremity	Fracture of humerus
	    Upper end, closed or open (812.0, 812.1)
	    Shaft or unspecified part, closed or open (812.2, 812.3)
	    Lower end, closed or open (812.4, 812.5)
	Fracture of radius and ulna
	    Upper end, closed or open (813.0, 813.1)
	    Shaft, open (813.3)
	    Lower end, closed or open (813.4, 813.5)
	    Unspecified part, closed or open (813.8, 813.9)

	Open wound of shoulder and upper arm
	    Complicated (880.1)
	    With tendon involvement (880.2)

	Open wound of elbow, forearm, and wrist
	    With tendon involvement (881.0)
	    Complicated (881.2)

	Traumatic amputation of
	    Thumb (complete) (partial) (885)
	    Other finger(s) (complete) (partial) (886)
	    Arm and hand (complete) (partial) (unilateral, below elbow, without mention of complication) (887.0)
	    Arm and hand (complete) (partial) (unilateral, below elbow, complicated) (887.1)
	    Arm and hand (complete) (partial) (unilateral, at or above elbow, without mention of complication) (887.2)
	    Arm and hand (complete) (partial) (unilateral, at or above elbow, complicated) (887.3)

	Crushing injury of
	    Upper limb (shoulder and upper arm) (927.0)
	    Upper limb (elbow and forearm) (927.1)
	    Upper limb (wrist and hand[s]) (927.2)
	    Upper limb (finger) (927.3)
	    Upper limb (multiple sites) (927.8)

	Burn of
	    Upper limb, except wrist and hand (943)
	    Wrist(s) and hand(s) (944)

	Injury to peripheral nerve(s) of shoulder girdle and upper limb (955)
Low back	Lumbar spondylosis with myelopathy (721.4)
	Lumbar intervertebral disc disorder with myelopathy (725.73)
	Disorders of sacrum (742.6)
	Other unspecified back disorders (724.9)
	Spondylolisthesis (756.12)

	Fracture of vertebral column with spinal cord injury
	    Lumbar, closed (806.4)
	    Lumbar, open (806.5)
	    Sacrum and coccyx, closed (806.6)
	    Sacrum and coccyx, open (806.7)

	Spinal cord injury without evidence of spinal bone injury (sacral) (952.2)

Note. Numbers in parentheses are codes from the *International Classification of Diseases, Ninth Revision, Clinical Modification* (*ICD-9-CM;* American Medical Association, 2008).

Table F2. Factors Affecting Utilization of Occupational Therapy Services

Factors That Increase Utilization	Factors That Reduce Utilization
Service Delivery or System Factors	
Delay in authorization for orthosis	Preoperative education or instruction
Intensity of work (heavy construction labor or meat packing vs. light office work)	Preoperative application of orthotics
	Presurgical occupational therapy treatment
Person Factors	
Multiple surgical procedures	
Type of surgery	
Surgeries that have a cumulative cause (vs. a traumatic cause)	
Infection	
Difficult scar management	
Edema	
Existing comorbidities (e.g., diabetes, cardiac or pulmonary condition, arthritis, renal disease)	
Complicating health behavior factors (e.g., smoking, high alcohol intake)	
Poor motivation	
Poor attendance	
Limited cognitive abilities	
Socioeconomic factors (person and environmental)	

suggested by therapists participating in a TriHealth Corporate Health services study of data from the Focus on Therapeutic Outcomes network (Linz et al., 2002). This survey, like ours, suggests that therapy initiated soon after the injury or referral, patient education, and patient participation (e.g., compliance with home exercise program) are all factors in improving outcomes. Many therapists pointed to the role of good communication among physicians and other members of the health care team in positive outcomes with decreased utilization.

Factors that most likely to *increase* utilization of occupational therapy (often/always >60%) include the following:

- Longer-than-average length of time between injury and surgery, with no therapy intervention
- Longer-than-recommended length of time between injury and of start of occupational therapy (e.g., delays in referrals, delays in insurance authorization)
- Multiple surgical procedures
- Nerve involvement
- Slow wound healing
- Complex injury

- Continued pain or joint stiffness
- Patient noncompliance (e.g., with home program, wound care).

Factors most likely to *reduce* utilization of occupational therapy (often/always >60%) include the following:

- Timely start of occupational therapy services
- Ergonomic intervention programs in the workplace
- Activity analysis resulting in job modification
- Compliance with intervention instructions and home exercise program
- Compliance with precautions
- Consistent attendance
- Good mental attitude toward return to work
- Good support by family, coworkers, and friends.

Orthotics Management

Orthotics fabrication, fitting, and training are important areas of occupational therapy practice, especially with upper extremity injuries. Early application of an orthotic, when indicated, and proper fitting can help clients resume normal activities and achieve return-to-work goals earlier. For that reason, therapists participating in the upper extremity survey were asked to indicate those conditions for which a custom-fabricated, custom-fitted, or modified off-the-shelf orthotic would usually be included in the plan of treatment. Based on diagnosis alone, more than 70% of the therapists interviewed indicated that orthotics would likely be part of the occupational therapy care plan for upper limb crushing injuries; burns; fractures; dislocations; mononeuritis; sprains and strains; and other disorders of synovium, tendon, and bursa.

Conclusion

For occupational therapy clients with work-related injuries and illnesses, rate of improvement and the capability to return to work vary widely depending on an array of considerations, including intrinsic client factors and contexts and extrinsic environmental factors related to the features and demands of the job. Each factor affects outcomes to some degree, depending on a specific case situation.

■ ■ ■

Appendix G.
Selected *CPT*^{TM} Coding for Occupational Therapy Evaluations and Interventions

The following chart can assist occupational therapy practitioners in making clinically appropriate decisions in selecting the most relevant *Current Procedural Terminology*^{TM} *(CPT)* code to describe occupational therapy evaluation and intervention. Occupational therapy practitioners should use the most appropriate code from the current *CPT* based on specific services provided, individual client goals, payer policy, and common usage.

Examples of Occupational Therapy Evaluations and Interventions	Suggested *CPT*^{TM} Code(s)
Evaluation	
■ Develop occupational profile ■ Analyze occupational performance	97003—Occupational therapy evaluation 97004—Occupational therapy reevaluation
■ Administer specific performance tests ■ Administer functional capacity evaluation (FCE)	97750—Physical performance test or measurement (e.g., musculoskeletal, functional capacity), with written report, each 15 min
■ Assess need for, design, and fabricate an orthotic to support the wrist to overcome weakness and allow client to maintain hand in proper position to resume daily activities ■ Fit orthotic to body, train in proper care, and develop daily wear-time schedule ■ Refer to Medicare National Level II Healthcare Common Procedure Coding System codes for billing actual orthosis (http://www.cms.hhs.gov/hcpcsreleasecodesets/).	97760—Orthotic(s) management and training (including assessment and fitting when not otherwise reported), upper extremity(s), lower extremity(s), and/or trunk, each 15 min
■ Modify orthotic to avoid skin irritation and assess use in performance (e.g., ability to type)	97762—Checkout for orthotic or prosthetic use, established patient, each 15 min
■ Assess client requirements for specialized mobility equipment, such as powered wheelchairs, to enable community and work participation ■ Observe client in workplace environment and recommend safe methods of operating wheelchair at work	97542—Wheelchair management (e.g., assessment, fitting, training), each 15 min
■ Provide functional exercises to increase range of motion, strength, and mobility to enable increased participation in required work tasks	97110—Therapeutic procedure, one or more areas, each 15 min; therapeutic exercises to develop strength and endurance, range of motion, and flexibility 97113—Aquatic therapy with therapeutic exercises
■ Design graded tasks to increase coordination and balance needed to perform work activities, such as climbing ladders ■ Provide graded keyboard activities to facilitate speed and fine motor coordination of fingers commensurate with requirements for client's return to full-time secretarial position	97112—Therapeutic procedure, one or more areas, each 15 min; neuromuscular reeducation of movement, balance, coordination, kinesthetic sense, posture, and/or proprioception for sitting and/or standing activities

(continued)

Examples of Occupational Therapy Evaluations and Interventions	Suggested *CPT*™ Code(s)
■ Train in use of memory exercises to enhance client's ability to remember information necessary to return to work (e.g., inventory numbers, e-mail addresses) ■ Teach sensory focus as a pain control technique	97532—Development of cognitive skills to improve attention, memory, and problem solving (includes compensatory training); direct (one-on-one) patient contact by the provider, each 15 min
■ Provide direct treatment to facilitate dynamic work simulated activities to increase functional performance—for example, climbing ladders; gear shifting; simulated lifting, pushing, and pulling; materials handling—with goal of integrating learned body mechanics into job task ■ Provide strengthening activities, incorporating safe lifting techniques, to facilitate bending, lifting, and carrying > 80-lb cartons	97530—Therapeutic activities; direct (one-on-one) patient contact by the provider (use of dynamic activities to improve functional performance), each 15 min
■ Teach adapted techniques to perform basic self-care activities as well as meal preparation during immobilization period immediately following hand surgery ■ Design and observe behavioral-oriented graded activity focusing on resuming normal basic and instrumental activities of daily living with goal of return to work or to progress to work reconditioning and work hardening activities	97535—Self-care/home management training (e.g., activities of daily living and compensatory training, meal preparation, safety procedures, instruction in use of assistive technology devices/adaptive equipment); direct (one-on-one) contact by the provider, each 15 min
■ Conduct work site visit, including a functional job analysis and ergonomic evaluation, with modifications made including use of hand truck for material handling and incorporation of rest and stretch breaks during work routine ■ Teach energy conservation techniques to facilitate successful return to work ■ Initiate work modifications—for example, changing to a lighter weight shovel, allowing for rest and stretch breaks, changing the movement pattern for shoveling from the truck, and rotating workers between tasks	97537—Community/work reintegration training (e.g., shopping, transportation, money management, avocational activities and/or work environment/ modification analysis, work task analysis, use of assistive technology device/ adaptive equipment), direct one-on-one contact by the provider, each 15 min
■ Apply physical agent modalities (e.g., fluidotherapy, ultrasound) to decrease pain, stiffness, and disuse of hand before engagement in treatment activities	97010-97039—Any physical agent applied to produce therapeutic changes to biologic tissue; includes but not limited to thermal, acoustic, light, mechanical, or electric energy
■ Apply pulsed ultrasound during active treatment sessions as a means of decreasing pain and discomfort over the lateral epicondyle and radial head	97035—Application of a modality to one or more areas; ultrasound, each 15 minutes
■ Provide joint mobilization to the wrist and fingers to maintain joint play and joint integrity to enable client to safely grasp tools, writing utensils, and other items	97140—Manual therapy techniques (e.g., mobilization/manipulation, manual lymphatic drainage, manual traction), one or more regions, each 15 min
■ Provide a work conditioning program that includes (a) intense (3–4 hours) activities designed to improve flexibility, mobility, pain control, conditioning, endurance, aerobic fitness, and strength related to work activities and (b) use of daily modalities for symptom control before participation in work-related exercise and activities, as needed ■ Provide a work hardening program that includes (a) work capacity evaluation, (b) intense (4-8-hr, 5-day-a-week) program of real and simulated work and functional activities to prepare client for return to a specific job, and (c) a functional capacity evaluation to definitively ascertain the client's ability to return to work	97545—Work hardening/conditioning; initial 2 hr 97546—Work hardening/conditioning; each additional hour

Note. The *CPT* codes referenced in this document do not represent all of the possible codes that may be used in occupational therapy evaluation and intervention. Not all payers will reimburse for all codes. Refer to the most current *CPT* for the complete list of available codes.

CPT™ is a trademark of the American Medical Association (AMA). *CPT* five-digit codes, nomenclature, and other data are copyright 2008 by the American Medical Association. All Rights Reserved. No fee schedules, basic units, relative values, or related listings are included in *CPT*. The AMA assumes no liability for the data contained herein.

Codes shown refer to *CPT 2009*. *CPT* codes are updated annually. New and revised codes become effective January 1. Always refer to the annual updated *CPT* publication for the most current codes.

Individuals With Work-Related Injuries and Illnesses

Appendix H. Preparation and Qualifications of Occupational Therapists and Occupational Therapy Assistants

Who Are Occupational Therapists?

To practice as an occupational therapist, the individual trained in the United States

- Has graduated from an occupational therapy program accredited by the Accreditation Council for Occupational Therapy Education (ACOTE®) or predecessor organizations;
- Has successfully completed a period of supervised fieldwork experience required by the recognized educational institution where the applicant met the academic requirements of an educational program for occupational therapists that is accredited by ACOTE or predecessor organizations;
- Has passed a nationally recognized entry-level examination for occupational therapists; and
- Fulfills state requirements for licensure, certification, or registration.

Educational Programs for the Occupational Therapist

These include the following:
- Biological, physical, social, and behavioral sciences
- Basic tenets of occupational therapy
- Occupational therapy theoretical perspectives
- Screening and evaluation

- Formulation and implementation of an intervention plan
- Context of service delivery
- Management of occupational therapy services (master's level)
- Leadership and management (doctoral level)
- Use of research
- Professional ethics, values, and responsibilities.

The fieldwork component of the program is designed to develop competent, entry-level, generalist occupational therapists by providing experience with a variety of clients across the life span and in a variety of settings. Fieldwork is integral to the program's curriculum design and includes an in-depth experience in delivering occupational therapy services to clients, focusing on the application of purposeful and meaningful occupation and/or research, administration, and management of occupational therapy services.

The fieldwork experience is designed to promote clinical reasoning and reflective practice, to transmit the values and beliefs that enable ethical practice, and to develop professionalism and competence in career responsibilities. Doctoral-level students must also complete a doctoral experiential component designed to develop advanced skills beyond a generalist level.

Who Are Occupational Therapy Assistants?

To practice as an occupational therapy assistant, the individual trained in the United States

- Has graduated from an occupational therapy assistant program accredited by ACOTE or predecessor organizations;
- Has successfully completed a period of supervised fieldwork experience required by the recognized educational institution where the applicant met the academic requirements of an educational program for occupational therapy assistants that is accredited by ACOTE or predecessor organizations;
- Has passed a nationally recognized entry-level examination for occupational therapy assistants; and
- Fulfills state requirements for licensure, certification, or registration.

Educational Programs for the Occupational Therapy Assistant

These include the following:

- Biological, physical, social, and behavioral sciences
- Basic tenets of occupational therapy
- Screening and assessment
- Intervention and implementation
- Context of service delivery
- Assistance in management of occupational therapy services

- Professional literature
- Professional ethics, values, and responsibilities.

The fieldwork component of the program is designed to develop competent, entry-level, generalist occupational therapy assistants by providing experience with a variety of clients across the life span and in a variety of settings. Fieldwork is integral to the program's curriculum design and includes an in-depth experience in delivering occupational therapy services to clients, focusing on the application of purposeful and meaningful occupation. The fieldwork experience is designed to promote clinical reasoning appropriate to the occupational therapy assistant role, to transmit the values and beliefs that enable ethical practice, and to develop professionalism and competence in career responsibilities.

Regulation of Occupational Therapy Practice

All occupational therapists and occupational therapy assistants must practice under federal and state law. Currently, 50 states, the District of Columbia, Puerto Rico, and Guam have enacted laws regulating the practice of occupational therapy.

Note. The majority of this information is taken from the *Accreditation Standards for a Doctoral-Degree-Level Educational Program for the Occupational Therapist* (AOTA, 2007a), *Accreditation Standards for a Master's-Degree-Level Educational Program for the Occupational Therapist* (AOTA, 2007b), and *Accreditation Standards for an Educational Program for the Occupational Therapy Assistant* (AOTA, 2007c).

■ ■ ■

References

ACGIH Worldwide. (2002). *Threshold limit value for chemical substances and physical agents and biological exposure indices.* Cincinnati, OH: Author.

Agency on Healthcare Research and Quality. (n.d.). *Standard recommendation language.* Retrieved on March 6, 2009, from http://www.ahrq.gov/clinic/uspstf/standard.htm.

American Alliance for Health, Physical Education, Recreation, and Dance. (1988). *Physical best: A physical fitness education and assessment program.* Reston, VA: Author.

American Educational Research Association, American Psychological Association, & National Council on Measurement in Education. (1999). *Standards for educational and psychological testing.* Washington, DC: Authors.

American Medical Association. (2008). *International classification of diseases, ninth revision, clinical modification (ICD-9-CM;* Hospital, Vols. 1–3). Chicago: Author.

American Occupational Therapy Association. (1979). *Occupational therapy product output reporting system and uniform terminology for reporting occupational therapy services.* (Available from American Occupational Therapy Association, 4720 Montgomery Lane, Bethesda, MD 20814)

American Occupational Therapy Association. (1989). *Uniform terminology for occupational therapy* (2nd ed.). (Available from American Occupational Therapy Association, 4720 Montgomery Lane, Bethesda, MD 20814)

American Occupational Therapy Association. (1994). Uniform terminology for occupational therapy (3rd ed.). *American Journal of Occupational Therapy, 48,* 1047–1054.

American Occupational Therapy Association. (2002). Occupational therapy practice framework: Domain and process. *American Journal of Occupational Therapy, 56,* 609–639.

American Occupational Therapy Association. (2005). Standards of practice for occupational therapy. *American Journal of Occupational Therapy, 59,* 663–665.

American Occupational Therapy Association. (2006). Policy 1.44: Categories of occupational therapy personnel. In *Policy manual* (pp. 33–34). Bethesda, MD: Author.

American Occupational Therapy Association. (2007a). Accreditation standards for a doctoral-degree-level educational program for the occupational therapist. *American Journal of Occupational Therapy, 61,* 641–651.

American Occupational Therapy Association. (2007b). Accreditation standards for a master's-degree-level educational program for the occupational therapist. *American Journal of Occupational Therapy, 61,* 652–661.

American Occupational Therapy Association. (2007c). Accreditation standards for an educational program for the occupational therapy assistant. *American Journal of Occupational Therapy, 61,* 686–700.

American Occupational Therapy Association. (2008a). Guidelines for documentation of occupational therapy. *American Journal of Occupational Therapy, 62,* 684–690.

American Occupational Therapy Association. (2008b). Occupational therapy practice framework: Domain and process (2nd ed.). *American Journal of Occupational Therapy, 62,* 625–683.

American Occupational Therapy Association. (2009). Guidelines for supervision, roles, and responsibilities during the delivery of occupational therapy services. *American Journal of Occupational Therapy, 63.*

American Thoracic Society. (2002). ATS statement: Guidelines for the six-minute walk test. *American Journal Respiratory and Critical Care Medicine, 166*(1), 111–117.

Americans With Disabilities Act of 1990. P. L. 101-336.

Ashworth, B. (1964). Preliminary trial of carisoprodal in multiple sclerosis. *Practitioner, 192,* 540–542.

Baum, C., Morrison, T., Hahn, M., & Edwards, D. (2003, 2008). *Executive function performance test: Test protocol booklet. Program in occupational therapy.* St. Louis, MO: Washington University School of Medicine. (Available from baumc@wustl.edu)

Beck, A. T., Rial, W. Y., & Rickets K. (1974). Short form of depression inventory: Cross-validation. *Psychological Reports, 34*(3), 1184–1186.

Beck, A. T., Ward, C. H., Mendelson, M., Mock, J., & Erbaugh, J. (1961). An inventory for measuring depression. *Archives of General Psychiatry 4,* 561–571.

Bekkering, G., van Tulder, M., Hendriks, E., Koopmanschap, M., Knol, D., Bouter, L., et al. (2005). Implementation of clinical guidelines on physical therapy for patients with low back pain: Randomized trial comparing patient outcomes after a standard and active implementation strategy. *Journal of Physical Therapy, 85,* 544–555.

Belza, B., Henke, C., Yelin, E., Epstein, W., & Gilliss, C. (1993). Correlates of fatigue in older adults with rheumatoid arthritis. *Nursing Research, 42*(2), 93–99.

Bennett, G. K. (1985). *Bennett Hand–Tool Dexterity Test.* San Antonio, TX: Pearson.

Berg, K., Wood-Dauphinee, S., & Williams, J. (1995). The Balance Scale: Reliability assessment with elderly residents and patients with an acute stroke. *Scandinavian Journal of Rehabilitation Medicine, 27*(1), 27–36.

Bingol, U., Altan, L., & Yurtkuran, M. (2005). Low-power laser treatment for shoulder pain. *Photomedicine and Laser Surgery, 23,* 459–464.

Bisset, L., Paungmali, A., Vicenzino, B., & Beller, E. (2005). A systematic review and meta-analysis of clinical trials on physical interventions for lateral epicondylalgia. *British Journal of Sports Medicine, 39,* 411–422.

Bleakley, C., McDonough, S., & MacAuley, D. (2004). The use of ice in the treatment of acute soft-tissue injury: A systematic review of randomized controlled trials. *American Journal of Sports Medicine, 32,* 251–261.

Borg, G. (1990). Psychophysical scaling with applications in physical work and the perception of exertion. *Scandinavian Journal of Work, Environment, and Health, 16*(1), 55–58.

Borkholder, C. D., Hill, V. A., & Fess, E. E. (2004). The efficacy of splinting for lateral epicondylitis: A systematic review. *Journal of Hand Therapy, 17,* 181–199.

Brosseau, L., Casimiro, L., Milne, S., Robinson, V. A., Shea, B. J., Tugwell, P., et al. (2002). Deep transverse friction massage for treating tendonitis. *Cochrane Database of Systematic Reviews, 4,* CD003528.

Brosseau, L., MacLeay, L., Robinson, V. A., Tugwell, P., & Wells, G. (2003). Intensity of exercise for the treatment of osteoarthritis. *Cochrane Database of Systematic Reviews, 2,* CD004259.

Brosseau, L., Robinson, V., Wells, G., deBie, R., Gam, A., Harman, K., et al. (2004). Low level laser therapy (Classes I, II, and III) for treating osteoarthritis. *Cochrane Database of Systematic Reviews, 3,* CD002046.

Brubaker, P., Fearon, F., Smith, S. M., McKibbin, R., J., Alday, J., Andrews, S. S., et al. (2007). Sensitivity and specificity of the Blankenship FCE system's indicators of submaximal effort. *Journal of Orthopaedic and Sports Physical Therapy, 37*(4), 161–168.

Callinan, N., McPherson, S., Cleaveland, S., Voss, D., Rainville, D., & Tokar, N. (2003). Effectiveness of hydroplasty and therapeutic exercise for treatment of frozen shoulder. *Journal of Hand Therapy, 16,* 219–224.

Case-Smith, J. (2003). Outcomes in hand rehabilitation using occupational therapy services. *American Journal of Occupational Therapy, 57,* 499–506.

Cawley, J. (2000). An instrumental variables approach to measuring the effect of body weight on employment disability. *Health Services Research, 35,* 1159–1179.

Centers for Disease Control and Prevention. (2001). Nonfatal occupational injuries and illnesses treated in hospital emergency departments—United States 1998. *Morbidity and Mortality Weekly Report, 50,* 313–317.

Cipriany-Dacko, L., Innerst, D., Johannsen, J., & Rude, V. (1997). Interrater reliability of the Tinetti balance scores in novice and experienced physical therapy clinicians. *Archives of Physical Medicine and Rehabilitation, 78,* 1160–1164.

Crawford J., & Crawford, D. (1956). *Crawford Small Parts Dexterity Test.* San Antonio, TX: Psychological Corporation.

Daltroy, L., Iverson, M., Larson, M., Lew, R., Wright, E., Ryan, J., et al. (1997). A controlled trial of an educational program to prevent low back injuries. *New England Journal of Medicine, 337*(5), 322–328.

de Croon, E., Sluiter, J., & Frings-Dresen, M. (2003). Need for recovery after work predicts sickness absence: A 2-year prospective cohort study in truck drivers. *Journal of Psychosomatic Research, 55,* 331–339.

Denniston, P. L. (2008). *Official disability guidelines* (ODG: Treatment in Workers' Compensation). Retrieved February 2, 2009, from http://www.disability-durations.com

Derebery, V. J., Devenport, J. N., Giang, G. M., & Fogarty, W. T. (2005). The effects of splinting on outcomes for epicondylitis. *Archives of Physical Medicine and Rehabilitation, 86,* 1081–1088.

Derogatis, L. (1977). *Symptom Checklist 90: Pearson assessments for educational, clinical, and psychological use.* Bloomington, MN: Pearson Education.

Diercks, R. L., & Stevens, M. (2004). Gentle thawing of the frozen shoulder: A prospective study of supervised neglect versus intensive physical therapy in seventy-seven patients with frozen shoulder syndrome followed up for two years. *Journal of Shoulder and Elbow Surgery, 13,* 499–502.

Dodrill, C. (1983). Long-term reliability of the Wonderlic Personnel Test. *Journal of Consulting and Clinical Psychology, 51,* 316–317.

Dunn, W., Brown, C., & McGuigan, A. (1994). The ecology of human performance: A framework for considering the effect of context. *American Journal of Occupational Therapy, 48,* 595–607.

Dunn, W., McClain, L. H., Brown, C., & Youngstrom, M. J. (1998). The ecology of human performance. In M. E. Neistadt & E. B. Crepeau (Eds.), *Willard and Spackman's occupational therapy* (9th ed., pp. 525–535). Philadelphia: Lippincott Williams & Wilkins.

Dworking, S., Sherman, J., Mancl, L., Ohrbach, R., Leresche, L., & Truelove, E. (2002). Reliability, validity, and clinical utility of the research diagnostic criteria for temporomandibular disorders axis II scales: Depression, non-specific physical symptoms, and graded chronic pain. *Journal of Orofacial Pain, 16,* 207–220.

Egan, M. Y., & Brosseau, L. (2007). Splinting for osteoarthritis of the carpometacarpal joint: A review of the evidence. *American Journal of Occupational Therapy, 61,* 70–78.

Ejnisman, B., Andreoli, C. V., Soares, B. G. O., Fallopa, F., Peccin, M. S., Abdalla, R. J., et al.

(2005). Interventions for tears of the rotator cuff in adults. *Cochrane Database of Systematic Reviews, 1,* CD002758.

Engel, J. (2006). Evaluation and pain management. In H. Pendleton & W. Schultz-Krohn (Eds.), *Pedretti's occupational therapy practice skills for physical dysfunction* (6th ed., pp. 646–655). St. Louis, MO: Elsevier/Mosby.

Fairbank, J. C. T., Couper J., Davies, J. B., & O'Brien, J. P. (1980). The Oswestry Low Back Pain Disability Questionnaire. *Physiotherapy, 66*(8), 271–273.

Fairbank, J., Frost, H., Wilson-MacDonald, J., Yu, L. M., Barker, K., & Collins, R. [Spine Stabilisation Group]. (2005). Randomised controlled trial to compare surgical stabilisation of the lumbar spine with an intensive rehabilitation programme for patients with chronic low back pain: The MRC spine stabilisation trial. *British Medical Journal, 330*(7502), 1233.

Feehan, L., & Bassett, K. (2004). Is there evidence for early mobilization following an extraarticular hand fracture? *Journal of Hand Therapy, 17,* 300–308.

Feldt, K. (2000). The checklist of nonverbal pain indicators. *Pain Management Nursing, 1*(1), 13–21.

Feuerstein, M., Berkowitz, S., & Huang, G. (1999). Predictors of occupational low back disability: Implications for secondary prevention. *Journal of Occupational and Environmental Medicine, 41,* 1024–1031.

Field, H., Bayley, G., & Bayley, S. (1977). Employment test validation for minority production workers. *Personnel Psychology, 30*(1), 37–46. (Assessment available from Harcourt Assessments, San Antonio, TX)

Field, T., Peck, M., Hernandez-Reif, M., Krugman, S., Burman, I., & Ozment-Schenck, L. (2000). Postburn itching, pain, and psychological symptoms are reduced with massage therapy. *Journal of Burn Care and Rehabilitation, 21,* 189–193.

Filiz, M., Cakmak, A., & Ozcan, E. (2005). The effectiveness of exercise programmes after lumbar disc surgery: A randomized controlled study. *Clinical Rehabilitation, 19,* 4–11.

Fleishman, E., & Hempel, W. (1954). A factor analysis of dexterity tests. *Personnel Psychology, 7*(1), 15–32.

French, S., Cameron, M., Walker, B., Reggars, J., & Esterman, A. (2006). Superficial heat or cold for low back pain. *Cochrane Database of Systematic Reviews, 3,* CD004750.

Fritz, J., Delitto, A., & Erhard, R. (2003). Comparison of classification-based physical therapy with therapy based on clinical practice guidelines for patients with acute low back pain. *Spine, 28,* 1363–1371.

Functional Assessment Network. (2003). *A systematic approach for a functional assessment process: Guidelines for injured workers.* Retrieved March 4, 2009, from http://www.fhs.mcmaster.ca/rehab/FA%20Guidelines.pdf

Gage, M., Noh, S., Polatajko, H., & Kasper, V. (1994). Measuring perceived self-efficacy in occupational therapy. *American Journal of Occupational Therapy, 48,* 783–790.

Garner, L. (2005, June). Guide to hand protection. *Occupational Health and Safety.* Retrieved June 30, 2007, from www.ohsonline.com/articles/44879

Ger, L., Ho, S., Sun, S., Wang, M., & Cleeland, C. S. (1999). Validation of the Brief Pain Inventory in a Taiwanese population. *Journal of Pain and Symptom Management, 18,* 316–322.

Geraets, J. J. X. R., Goossens, M. E. J. B., de Groot, I. J. M., de Bruijn, C. P. C., de Bie, R. B., Dinant, G.-J., et al. (2005). Effectiveness of a graded exercise therapy program for patients with chronic shoulder complaints. *Australian Journal of Physiotherapy, 51,* 87–94.

Gibson, K., Growse, A., Korda, L., Wray, E., & MacDermid, J. C. (2004). The effectiveness of rehabilitation for nonoperative management of shoulder instability: A systematic review. *Journal of Hand Therapy, 17,* 229–242.

Gibson, L., Strong, L., & Wallace, B. (2005). Functional capacity evaluation as a performance measure: Evidence for a new approach for clients with chronic back pain. *Clinical Journal of Pain, 21,* 207–215.

Gilworth, G., Chamberlain, M., Harvey, A., Woodhouse, A., Smith, J., Smyth, M. G., et al. (2003). Development of a work instability scale for rheumatoid arthritis. *Arthritis and Rheumatism, 49*(3), 349–354.

Glass, L. S. (Ed.). (2004). *Occupational medicine practice guidelines* (2nd ed.). Beverly Farms, MA: OEM Press.

Gloss, D., & Wardle, M. (1982). Use of the Minnesota Rate of Manipulation Test for disability evaluation. *Perceptual and Motor Skills, 55,* 527–532. (Assessment available from Lafayette Instrument Company, Lafayette, IN)

Golding, L. (Ed.). (2000). *The YMCA fitness testing and assessment manual* (4th ed.). Champaign, IL: Human Kinetics.

Grangaard, L. (2006). Low back pain. In H. M. Pendleton & W. Schultz-Krohn (Eds.), *Pedretti's occupational therapy: Practice skills for physical dysfunction* (6th ed., pp. 1036–1055). St. Louis, MO: Elsevier/Mosby.

Grant, H. J., Arthur, A., & Pichora, D. R. (2004). Evaluation of interventions for rotator cuff pathology: A systematic review. *Journal of Hand Therapy, 17,* 274–299.

Green, S., Buchbinder, R., & Hetrick, S. (2003). Physiotherapy interventions for shoulder pain. *Cochrane Database of Systematic Reviews, 2,* CD004258.

Green, S. E., Buchbinder, R., Forbes, A., & Glazier, R. (2006). Interventions for shoulder pain. *Cochrane Database of Systematic Reviews, 4,* CD001156.

Griffiths, A., Cox, T., Karanika, M., Khan, S., & Tomas, J. M. (2006). Work design and management in the manufacturing sector: Development and validation of the Work Organisation Assessment Questionnaire. *Occupational and Environmental Medicine, 63,* 669–675.

Gross, D. P., & Battié, M. C. (2003). Construct validity of a kinesiophysical functional capacity evaluation administered within a worker's compensation environment. *Journal of Occupational Rehabilitation, 13,* 287–295.

Gross, D. P., Battié, M. C., & Cassidy, J. D. (2004). The prognostic value of functional capacity evaluation in patients with chronic low back pain: Part 1. Timely return to work. *Spine, 29,* 914–919.

Guerriero, R., Rajwani, M., Gray, E., Platnick, H., & Da Re, R. (1999). A retrospective study of the effectiveness of physical rehabilitation of low back pain patients in a multidisciplinary setting. *Journal of the Canadian Chiropractic Association, 43*(2), 89–104.

Guler-Uysal, F., & Kozanoglu, E. (2004). Comparison of the early response of two methods of rehabilitation in adhesive capsulitis. *Swiss Medical Weekly, 134,* 353–358.

Guzelkucuk, U., Duman, I., Taskaynatan, M., & Dincer, K. (2007). Comparison of therapeutic activities with therapeutic exercises in the rehabilitation of young adult patients with hand injuries. *Journal of Hand Surgery, 32,* 1429–1435.

Guzman, J., Esmail, R., Karjalainen, K., Malmivaara, A., Irvin, E., & Bombardier, C. (2001). Multidisciplinary rehabilitation for low back pain: A systematic review. *British Medical Journal, 322,* 1511–1516.

Hagen, K., Hilde, G., Jamtvedt, G., & Winnem, M. (2004). Bed rest for acute low-back pain and sciatica. *Cochrane Database of Systematic Reviews, 4,* CD001254.

Haldorsen, E. M., Grasdal, A. L., Skouen, J. S., Risa, A. E., Skronholm, K., & Ursin, H. (2002). Is there a right treatment for a particular patient group? Comparison of ordinary treatment, light multidisciplinary treatment, and extensive multidisciplinary treatment for long-term sick-listed employees with musculoskeletal pain. *Pain, 95,* 49–63.

Hamilton, M. (1969). Diagnosis and rating of anxiety. *British Journal of Psychiatry* [Special Publication], *3,* 76–89.

Handoll, H. H. G., & Almaiyah, M. A. (2004). Surgical versus non-surgical treatment for acute anterior shoulder dislocation. *Cochrane Database of Systematic Reviews, 1,* CD004325.

Handoll, H. H. G., Gibson, J. N. A., & Madhok, R. (2003). Interventions for treating proximal humerus fractures in adults. *Cochrane Database of Systematic Reviews, 4,* CD000434.

Handoll, H. H. G., Hanchard, N. C. A., Goodchild, L., & Feary, J. (2006). Conservative management following closed reduction of traumatic anterior dislocation of the shoulder. *Cochrane Database of Systematic Reviews, 1,* CD004962.

Harada, N., Chiu, V., & Stewart, A. (1999). Mobility-related function in older adults: Assessment with a 6-minute walk test. *Archives of Physical Medicine and Rehabilitation, 80,* 837–841.

Hayden, J., van Tulder, M., Malmivaara, A., & Koes, B. (2005). Meta-analysis: Exercise therapy for non-specific low back pain. *Annals of Internal Medicine, 142,* 765–775.

Haythornthwaite, J., Lawrence, J. W., & Fauerbach, J. A. (2001). Brief cognitive interventions for burn pain. *Annals of Behavioral Medicine, 23,* 42–49.

Hazard, R., Haugh, L., Reid, S., Preble, J. B., & McDonald, L. (1996). Early prediction of chronic disability after occupational low back injury. *Spine, 21,* 945–951.

Heymans, M., van Tulder, M., Esmail, R., Bombardier, C., & Koes, B. (2004). Back schools for non-specific low-back pain. *Cochrane Database of Systematic Reviews, 3,* CD000261.

Hignett S., & McAtamney L. (2000). Rapid Entire Body Assessment (REBA). *Applied Ergonomics, 31,* 201–205.

Howard, N., Spielholz, P., Bao, S., Silverstein, B., & Fan, Z. (2009). Reliabililty of an observational tool to assess the organization of work. *International Journal of Industrial Ergonomics, 39,* 260–266.

Hudak, P., Amadio, P., Bombardier, C., Beaton, D., Cole, D., Davis, A., et al. (1996). Development of an upper extremity outcome measure: The DASH (Disabilities of the Arm, Shoulder, and Head). *American Journal of Industrial Medicine, 29,* 602–608.

Hurwitz, E., Morgenstern, H., & Chiao, C. (2005). Effects of recreational physical activity and back exercises on low back pain and psychological distress: Findings from the UCLA low back pain study. *American Journal of Public Health, 95,* 1817–1824.

Innes, E. (2006). Reliability and validity of functional capacity evaluations: An update. *International Journal of Disability Management Research, 135,* 135–148.

Innes, E., & Straker, L. (2003). Reliability of work-related assessments. *Work, 13,* 107–124.

Jay, M. A., Lamb, J. M., Watson, R. L., Young, I. A., Fearon, F. J., Alday, J. M., et al. (2000). Sensitivity and specificity of the indicators of sincere effort of the EPIC Lift Capacity test on a previously injured population. *Spine, 25,* 1405–1412.

Jurgel, J., Rannama, L., Gapeyeva, H., Ereline, J., Kolts, I., & Paasuke, M. (2005). Shoulder function in patients with frozen shoulder before and after 4-week rehabilitation. *Medicina (Kaunas), 41,* 30–38.

Karasek, R., Brisson, C., Kawakami, N., Houtman, I., Bongers, P., & Amick, B. (1998). The Job Content Questionnaire (JCQ): An instrument for internationally comparative assessments of psychosocial job characteristics. *Journal of Occupational Health Psychology, 3,* 322–355.

Karazman, R., Kloimuller, I., Geissler, H., & Karazman-Morawetz, I. (1999). Effect typology and Work Ability Index: Evaluating the success of health promotion in elder workforce. *Experimental Aging Research, 25,* 313–321.

Karjalainen, K., Malmivaara, A., van Tulder, M., Roine, R., Jauhiainen, M., Hurri, H., et al. (2000). Biopsychosocial rehabilitation for upper limb repetitive strain injuries in working age adults. *Cochrane Database of Systematic Reviews, 3,* CD002269.

Karjalainen, K., Malmivaara, A., van Tulder, M., Roine, R., Jauhiainen, M., Hurri, H., et al. (2001). Multidisciplinary biopsychosocial rehabilitation for subacute low-back pain among working age adults. *Cochrane Database of Systemic Reviews, 3,* CD002193.

Karjalainen, K., Malmivaara, A., van Tulder, M., Roine, R., Jauhiainen, M., Hurri, H., et al. (2003). Multidisciplinary biopsychosocial rehabilitation for neck and shoulder pain in working-age adults. *Cochrane Database of Systematic Reviews, 2,* CD002194.

Kellor, M., Frost, J., Silberber, N., Iversen, I., & Cummings, R. (1971). Purdue pegboard examiner manual. *American Journal of Occupational Therapy, 25*(2), 77–83.

Keogh, J., Nuwayhid, I., Gordon, J., & Gucer, P. (2000). The impact of occupational injury on injured workers and family: Outcomes of upper extremity cumulative trauma disorders in Maryland workers. *American Journal of Industrial Medicine, 39,* 4998–5061.

Khadilkar, A., Milne, S., Brosseau, L., Robinson, V., Saginur, M., Shea, B., et al. (2005). Trancutaneous electrical nerve stimulation (TENS) for chronic low-back pain. *Cochrane Database of Systemic Reviews, 2005, 2,* CD003008.

Khadilkar, A., Odebiyi, D. O., Brosseau, L., & Wells, G. A. (2008). Transcutaneous electrical nerve stimulation (TENS) versus placebo for chronic low-back pain. *Cochrane Database of Systematic Reviews, 4,* CD003008.

Kline, G., Porcari, J. P., Hintermeister, R., Freedson, P. S., Ward, A., McCarron, R. F., et al. (1987). Estimation of VO2max from a one-mile track walk, gender, age, and body weight. *Medicine and Science in Sports and Exercise, 19,* 253.

Kopec, J., & Esdaile, J. (1998). Occupational role performance in persons with back pain. *Disability and Rehabilitation, 20,* 373–379.

Koumantakis, G., Watson, P., & Oldham, J. (2005). Trunk muscle stabilization training plus general exercise versus general exercise only: Randomized controlled trial of patients with recurrent low back pain. *Physical Therapy, 85,* 209–223.

Law, M. (Ed.). (2002). *Evidence-based rehabilitation: A guide to practice.* Thorofare, NJ: Slack.

Law, M., Baptiste, S., Carswell, A., McColl, M., Polatajko, H., & Pollock, N. (1998). *Canadian Occupational Performance Measure manual* (3rd ed.). Ottowa, ON: CAOT Publications.

Law, M., & Baum, C. (1998). Evidenced-based occupational therapy. *Canadian Journal of Occupational Therapy, 65,* 131–135.

Lawlis, G., Cuencas, R., Selby, D., & McCoy, C. E. (1989). The development of the Dallas Pain Questionnaire: An assessment of the impact of spinal pain on behavior. *Spine, 14,* 511–516.

Leavitt, F., & Sweet, J. (1986). Characteristics and frequency of malingering among patients with low back pain. *Pain, 25,* 357–364.

Legge, J., & Burgess-Limerick, R. (2007). Reliability of the JobFit System Pre-Employment Functional Assessment Tool. *Work, 28,* 299–312.

Lerner, D., Amick, B., Rogers, W., Malspeis, S., Bungay, K., & Cynn, D. (2001). The work limitations questionnaire. *Medical Care, 39*(1), 72–85.

Lerner, D., Malspeis, S., Rogers, B., & Amick, B. (1995). A national survey of limitations in ability to work using a new work role functioning questionnaire. *Quality of Life Research, 4*(5), 455.

Liberty Mutual. (2004). *Liberty mutual material handling guidelines.* Retrieved February 22, 2009, from http://libertymmhtables.libertymutual.com/CM_LMTablesWeb/pdf/LibertyMutualTables.pdf

L'Insalata, J. C., Warren, R. F., Cohen, S. B., Altchek, D. W., & Peterson, M. G. (1997). A self-administered questionnaire for assessment of symptoms and function of the shoulder. *Journal of Bone and Joint Surgery, 17,* 739–748.

Linz, D., Shepherd, C., Ford, L., Ringley, L., Klekamp, J., & Duncan, J. (2002). Effectiveness of occupational medicine center–based physical therapy. *Journal of Occupational Environmental Medicine, 44*, 48–53.

Ludewig, P. M., & Borstad, J. D. (2003). Effects of a home exercise programme on shoulder pain and functional status in construction workers. *Occupational and Environmental Medicine, 60*, 841–849.

Lundblad, I., Elert, J., & Gerdle, B. (1999). Randomized controlled trial of physiotherapy and Feldenkrais interventions in female workers with neck–shoulder complaints. *Journal of Occupational Rehabilitation, 9*, 179–194.

Lygren, H., Dragesund, T., Joensen, J., Ask, T., & Moe-Nilssen, R. (2005). Test–retest reliability of the Progressive Isoinertial Lifting Evaluation (PILE). *Spine, 30*, 1070–1074.

MacDermid, J., Turgeon, T., Richards, R., Beadle, M., & Roth, J. (1998). Patient rating of wrist pain and disability: A reliable and valid measurement tool. *Journal of Orthopaedic Trauma, 12*(8), 577–586.

Maher, C., & Bear-Lehman, J. (2008). Orthopaedic conditions. In M. V. Radomski & C. A. Trombly Latham (Eds.), *Occupational therapy for physical dysfunction* (6th ed., pp. 1106–1130). Baltimore: Lippincott Williams & Wilkins.

Manniche, C., Asmussen, K., Lauritsen, B., Vinterberg H., Kreiner S., & Jordan A. (1994). Low Back Pain Rating Scale: Validation of a tool for assessment of low back pain. *Pain, 57*, 317–326.

Marcotte, A., Barker, R., Joyce, M., Miller, N., & Cogburn, E. (1997). *Preventing work-related musculoskeletal illnesses through ergonomics: The Air Force PREMIER program: Vol. 2. Job requirements and physical demands survey methodology guide (Field Version).* San Bernardino, CA: Earth Technology Corporation.

Martinez-Silvestrini, J. A., Newcomer, K. L., Gay, R. E., Schaefer, M. P., Kortebein, P., & Arendt, K. W. (2005). Chronic lateral epicondylitis: Comparative effectiveness of a home exercise program including stretching alone versus stretching supplemented with

eccentric or concentric strengthening. *Journal of Hand Therapy, 18*, 411–419.

Matheson, L. (1996). Relationships among age, body weight, resting heart rate, and performance in a new test of lift capacity. *Journal of Occupational Rehabilitation, 6*, 225–237.

Matheson, L. (2003). Functional capacity evaluation. In G. Andersson, S. Demeter, & G. Smith (Eds.), *Disability evaluation* (2nd ed.). Chicago: Mosby.

Matheson, L., Kaskutas, V., & Mada, D. (2001). Development and construct validation of the Hand Function Sort. *Journal of Occupational Rehabilitation, 11*(2), 75–86.

Matheson, L. N., & Matheson, M. L. (1993). *Performance assessment and capacity testing spinal function sort: Rating of perceived capacity.* Wildwood, MO: Employment Potential Improvement Corporation.

Matheson, L. N., Matheson, M., & Grant, J. (1993). Development of a measure of perceived functional ability. *Journal of Occupational Rehabilitation, 3*(1), 15–30.

Matheson, L. N., Mooney, V., Grant J., Leggett S., & Kenny, K. (1996). Standardized evaluation of work capacity. *Journal of Back and Musculoskeletal Rehabilitation, 6*, 249–264.

Mathias, S., Nayak, U. S., & Isaacs, B. (1986). Balance in elderly patients: The "Get-Up and Go" Test. *Archives of Physical Medicine and Rehabilitation, 67*, 387–389.

Mathiowetz, V., Kashman, N., Volland, G., Weber, K., Dowe, M., & Rogers, S. (1985). Grip and pinch strength: Normative data for adults. *Archives of Physical Medicine and Rehabilitation, 66*, 69–72.

McAtamney, L., & Corlett, E. N. (1993). RULA: A survey method for the investigation of work-related upper-limb disorders. *Applied Ergonomics, 24*, 91–99.

Melzack, R. (1975). The McGill Pain Questionnaire: Major properties and scoring methods. *Pain, 1*, 277–299.

Meyer, K., Fransen, J., Huwiler, H., Uebelhart, D., & Klipstein, A. (2005). Feasibility and results of a randomized pilot-study of a work rehabilitation programme. *Journal of Back and Musculoskeletal Rehabilitation, 18,* 67–78.

Michener, L. A., Walsworth, M. K., & Burnet, E. N. (2004). Effectiveness of rehabilitation for patients with subacromial impingement syndrome: A systematic review. *Journal of Hand Therapy, 17,* 152–164.

Michlovitz, S., Harris, B., & Watkins, M. (2004). Therapy interventions for improving joint range of motion: A systematic review. *Journal of Hand Therapy, 17,* 118–131.

Michlovitz, S., Hun, L., Erasala, G. N., Hengehold, D. A., & Weingand, K. W. (2004). Continuous low-level heat wrap therapy is effective for treating wrist pain. *Archives of Physical Medicine and Rehabilitation, 85,* 1409–1416.

Moore J., & Garg, A. (1995). The Strain Index: A proposed method to analyze jobs for risk of distal upper extremity disorders. *American Industrial Hygiene Journal, 56*(5), 443–458.

Moos, R. (1988). *Life stressors and social resources inventory.* (Available from Psychological Assessment Resources, 16204 North Florida Avenue, Lutz, FL 33549)

Moos, R. (1994). *Work Environment Scale manual: Development, applications, research* (3rd ed.). Palo Alto, CA: Consulting Psychologists Press.

Morley, S., Eccleston, C., & Williams, A. (1998). Systematic review and meta-analysis of randomized controlled tirals of cognitive behavior therapy and behavior therapy for chronic pain in adults, excluding headache. *Pain, 80,* 1–13.

Moyers, P. A., & Dale, L. M. (2007). *The guide to occupational therapy practice* (2nd ed.). Bethesda, MD: AOTA Press.

Muller, M., Tsui, D., Schnurr, R., Biddulph-Deisroth, L., Hard, J., & MacDermid, J. C. (2004). Effectiveness of hand therapy interventions in primary management of carpal tunnel syndrome: A systematic review. *Journal of Hand Therapy, 17,* 210–228.

Musich, S., Napier, D., & Edington, D. W. (2001). The association of health risks with workers' compensation costs. *Journal of Occupational and Environmental Medicine, 43*(6), 534–541.

Nash, C. E., Mickan, M., Del Mar, C. B., & Glasziou, P. P. (2004). Resting injured limbs delays recovery: A systematic review. *Journal of Family Practice, 53,* 706–712.

National Committee on Vital and Health Statistics. (2002). *Classifying and reporting functional status.* (Report of the Subcommittee on Population). Retrieved February 8, 2009, from www.ncvhs.hhs.gov/010716rp.htm

National Institute for Occupational Safety and Health. (1981). *Work practices guide for manual lifting* (Report No. 81-122). Cincinnati, OH: Author.

National Institute of Occupational Safety and Health. (1994). *Applications manual for the revised NIOSH lifting equation* (NIOSH Publication No. 94-110). Cincinnati, OH: Author.

Ng, C., Ho, D., & Chow, S. (1999). The Moberg Pickup Test: Results of testing with a standard protocol. *Journal of Hand Therapy, 12,* 309–312.

Nicholas, M. (1994). *Pain Self Efficacy Questionnaire (PSEQ): Preliminary report.* St. Leonards, New South Wales, Australia: University of Sydney Pain Management and Research Centre, Royal North Shore Hospital.

Novak, C. B., Collins, E. D., & Mackinnon, S. E. (1995). Outcome following conservative management of thoracic outlet syndrome. *Journal of Hand Surgery, 20A,* 542–548.

O'Brien, L., & Pandit, A. (2006). Silicon gel sheeting for preventing and treating hypertrophic and keloid scars. *Cochrane Database of Systematic Reviews, 1,* CD003826.

Occupational Safety and Health Administration. (2000). *VDT workstation checklist*. Retrieved March 23, 2009, from http://www.clemson.edu/ces/departments/ie/documents/Kimbler/APPD-Z.pdf

O'Connor, D., Marshall, S., & Massy-Westropp, N. (2003). Non-surgical treatment (other than steroid injection) for carpal tunnel syndrome. *Cochrane Database of Systematic Reviews, 1*, CD003219.

Oerlemans, H. M., Goris, R. J. A., de Boo, T., & Oostendorp, R. A. (1999). Do physical therapy and occupational therapy reduce the impairment percentage in reflex sympathetic dystrophy? *American Journal of Physical Medicine and Rehabilitation, 78*, 533–539.

Ohnmeiss, D., Vanharanta, H., & Elholm, J. (1999). Relationship of pain drawings to invasive tests assessing intervertebral disc pathology. *European Spine Journal, 8*, 126–131.

Ostelo, R., van Tulder, M., Vlaeyen, J., Linton, S., Morley, S., & Assendelft, W. (2005). Behavioural treatment for chronic low-back pain. *Cochrane Database of Systematic Reviews, 4*, CD002014.

Oud, T., Beelen, A., Eijffinger, E., & Nollet, F. (2007). Sensory re-education after nerve injury of the upper limb: A systematic review. *Clinical Rehabilitation, 21*, 483–494.

Persinger, R., Foster, C., Gibson, M., Fater, D., & Porcari, J. (2004). Consistency of the Talk Test for exercise prescription. *Medicine and Science in Sports and Exercise, 36*, 1632–1636.

Piotte, F., Gravel, D., Moffet, H., Fliszar, E., Roy, A., Nadeau, S., et al. (2004). Effects of repeated distension arthrographies combined with a home exercise program among adults with idiopathic adhesive capsulitis of the shoulder. *American Journal of Physical Medicine and Rehabilitation, 83*, 537–546.

Pober, D., Freedson, P., Kline, G., McKinnis, K. G., & Rippe, J. M. (2002). Development and validation of a one-mile treadmill walk test to predict peak oxygen uptake in healthy adults ages 40 to 79 years. *Canadian Journal of Applied Physiology, 27*, 575–589.

Portney, L., & Watkins, M. (2008). *Foundations of clinical research: Applications to practice* (3rd ed.). Upper Saddle River, NJ: Prentice Hall.

Pransky, G., Feuerstein, M., Himmelstein, J., Katz, J., & Vickers-Lahti, M.(1997). Measuring functional outcomes in work-related upper extremity disorders: Development and validation of the Upper Extremity Function Scale. *Journal of Occupational and Environmental Medicine, 39*, 1195–1202.

Prezzia, C., & Denniston, P. (2001). The use of evidence-based duration guidelines. *Journal of Workers Compensation, 10*(4). Retrieved March 9, 2009, from http://www.odg-disability.com/Journal%20of%20Workers%20Comp.pdf

Prigatano, G., Altman, I., & O'Brien, K. (1990). Behavioral limitations that traumatic-brain-injured patients tend to underestimate. *Clinical Neuropsychologist, 4*, 163–176.

Prudential Fitnessgram. (1992). Dallas: Cooper Institute for Aerobics Research.

Radloff, L. (1977). The CES–D scale: A self-report depression scale for research in the general population. *Applied Psychological Measures, 1*, 385–401.

Randlov, A., Ostergaard, M., Manniche, C., Kryger, P., Jordan, A., Heegard, S., et al. (1998). Intensive dynamic training for females with chronic neck/shoulder pain: A randomized controlled trial. *Clinical Rehabilitation, 12*, 200–210.

Ransford, A. O., Cairns, D., & Mooney, V. (1976). The pain drawing as an aid to the psychological evaluation of patients with low-back pain. *Spine, 2*, 127–134.

Reed, P. (Ed.). (2005). *The medical disability advisor* (5th ed.). Westminster, CO: Reed Group.

Reilly, M., Zbrozek, A., & Dukes, E. (1993). The validity and reproducibility of a work productivity and activity impairment instrument. *Pharmacoeconomics, 14*(5), 353–365.

Reneman, M., Brouwer, S., Meinema, A., Dijkstra, P., Geertzen, J., & Groothoff, J. (2004). Test–retest reliability of the Isernhagen Work Systems Functional Capacity Evaluation in healthy adults. *Journal of Occupational Rehabilitation, 14,* 295–305.

Reneman, M. F., Dijkstra, P. U., Westmaas, M., & Göeken, L. N. H. (2002). Test–retest reliability of lifting and carrying in a 2-day functional capacity evaluation. *Journal of Occupational Rehabilitation, 12,* 269–275.

Reneman, M. F., Fokkens, A. S., Dijkstra, P. U., Geertzen, J. H. B., & Groothoff, J. W. (2005). Testing lifting capacity: Validity of determining effort level by means of observation. *Spine, 30*(2), E40–E46.

Richard, R. L., Miller, S. F., Finley, R. K., & Jones, L. M. (1987). Comparison of the effect of passive exercise v. static wrapping on finger range of motion in the burned hand. *Journal of Burn Care and Rehabilitation, 8,* 576–578.

Robertson, I. H., Ward, T., Ridgeway, V., & Nimmo-Smith, I. (1996). The structure of normal human attention: The Test of Everyday Attention. *Journal of the International Neuropsychological Society, 2,* 525–534. (Assessment available from Harcourt Assessment, San Antonio, TX)

Roland, M., & Morris, R. (1983). A study of the natural history of back pain: Part I. Development of a reliable and sensitive measure of disability in low-back pain. *Spine, 3,* 141–144.

Ruiz-Quintanilla, S., & England, G. (1996). How working is defined: Structure and stability. *Journal of Organizational Behavior, 17,* 515–540.

Ryans, I., Montgomery, A., Galway, R., Kernohan, W. G., & McKane, R. (2005). A randomized controlled trial of intra-articular triamcinolone and/or physiotherapy in shoulder capsulitis. *Rheumatology, 44,* 529–535.

Sackett, D. L., Rosenberg, W. M., Muir Gray, J. A., Haynes, R. B., & Richardson, W. S. (1996). Evidence-based medicine. What it is and what it isn't. *British Medical Journal, 312,* 71–72.

Schonstein, E., Kenny, D., Keating, J., & Koes, B. (2003). Work conditioning, work hardening, and functional restoration for workers with back and neck pain. *Cochrane Database of Systematic Reviews, 3,* CD001822.

Severens, J. L., Oerlemans, H. M., Weegels, A. J. P. G., van't Hof, M. A., Oostendorp, R. A. B., & Goris, R. J. A. (1999). Cost-effectiveness analysis of adjuvant physical or occupational therapy for patients with reflex sympathetic dystrophy. *Archives of Physical Medicine and Rehabilitation, 80,* 1038–1043.

Sherer, M., Bergloff, P., Boake, C., High, W., & Levin, E. (1998). The Awareness Questionnaire: Factor structure and internal consistency. *Brain Injury, 12,* 63–68.

Sjogren, T., Nissinen, K. J., Jarvenpaa, S. K., Ojanen, M. T., Vanharanta, H., & Malkia, E. A. (2005). Effects of a workplace physical exercise intervention on the intensity of headache and neck and shoulder symptoms and upper extremity muscular strength of office workers: A cluster randomized controlled crossover trial. *Pain, 116,* 119–128.

Smidt, N., Assendelft, W. J. J., Arola, H., Malmivaara, A., Green, S., Buchbinder, R., et al. (2003). Effectiveness of physiotherapy for lateral epicondylitis: A systematic review. *Annals of Medicine, 35,* 51–62.

Smith, D., McMurray, N., & Disler, P. (2002). Early intervention for acute back injury: Can we finally develop an evidence-based approach? *Clinical Rehabilitation, 16,* 1–11.

Soer, R., van der Schans, C., Groothoff, J., Geertzen, J. H., & Reneman, M. F. (2008). Towards consensus in operational definitions in functional capacity evaluation: A Delphi survey. *Journal of Occupational Rehabilitation, 18,* 389–400.

Solway S., Brooks D., Lacasse Y., & Thomas S. (2001). A qualitative systematic overview of the measurement properties of functional walk tests used in the cardiorespiratory domain. *Chest, 119*(1), 256–270.

Staal, J., Hlobil, H., Twisk, J., Smid, T., Köke, A., & van Mechelen, W. (2004). Graded activity for low back pain in occupational health care. *Annals of Internal Medicine, 140,* 77–85.

Stasinopoulos, D. I., & Johnson, J. I. (2005). Effectiveness of low-level laser therapy for lateral elbow tendinopathy. *Photomedicine and Laser Surgery, 23,* 425–430.

Struijs, P. A., Smidt, N. N., Arola, H., Van Dijk, C. N., Buchbinder, R., & Assendelft, W. J. J. (2002). Orthotic devices for the treatment of tennis elbow. *Cochrane Database of Systematic Reviews, 1,* CD001821.

Stutzman, L. (2001, August). Evidence-based return to work guidelines. *CWCE Magazine,* pp. 36–38.

Tait, R., Pollard, C., Margolis, R., Duckro, P. N., & Krause, S. J. (1987). The Pain Disability Index: Psychometric and validity data. *Archives of Physical Medicine and Rehabilitation, 68,* 438–441.

Tiffin, J. (1999). *Purdue pegboard* (rev. ed.). Lafayette, IN: Lafayette Instrument Company.

Trombly, C. A. (1995). Occupation: Purposefulness and meaningfulness as therapeutic mechanisms. *American Journal of Occupational Therapy, 56,* 250–259.

Trudel, D., Duley, J., Zastrow, I., Kerr, E. W., Davidson, R., & MacDermid, J. C. (2004). Rehabilitation for patients with lateral epicondylitis: A systematic review. *Journal of Hand Therapy, 17,* 243–266.

Tuckwell, N., Straker, L., & Barrett, T. (2002). Test–retest reliability on nine tasks of the Physical Work Performance Evaluation. *Work, 19,* 243–253.

Turner, J., Franklin, G., Fulton-Kehow, D., Sheppard, L., Wickizer, T., Wu, R., et al. (2007). Early predictors of chronic work disability associated with carpal tunnel syndrome: A longitudinal workers' compensation cohort study. *Americal Journal of Industrial Medicine, 50,* 498–506.

U.S. Bureau of Labor Statistics. (2008). Nonfatal occupational injuries and illnesses requiring days away from work, 2007 [Press release from the U.S. Department of Labor, No. 08-1716]. Washington, DC: Author.

U. S. Department of Labor. (1978). *Uniform guidelines for employee selection.* Retrieved March 3, 2009, from http://www.dol.gov/dol/allcfr/Title_41/Part_60-3/toc.htm

Van de Streek, M. D., van der Schans, C. P., de Greef, M. G. H., & Postema, K. (2004). The effect of a forearm/hand splint compared with an elbow band as a treatment for lateral epicondylitis. *Prosthetics and Orthotics International, 28,* 183–189.

van der Heijden, G. J. M. C., Leffers, P., & Bouter, L. M. (2000). Shoulder Disability Questionnaire design and responsiveness of functional status measure. *Journal of Clinical Epidemiology, 53,* 29–38.

van der Windt, D. A., van der Heijden, G. J., van den Berg, S. G., ter Riet, G., de Winter, A. F., & Bouter, L. M. (1999). Ultrasound therapy for musculoskeletal disorders: A systematic review. *Pain, 81,* 257–271.

Verhagen, A. P., Karels, C., Bierma-Zeinstra, S. M. A., Burdorf, L., Feleus, A., Dahaghin, S., et al. (2006). Ergonomic and physiotherapeutic interventions for treating work-related complaints of the arm, neck, or shoulder in adults. *Cochrane Database of Systematic Reviews, 3,* CD003471.

Vermeulen, H. M., Rozing, P. M., Obermann, W. R., le Cessie, S., & Vliet Vleland, T. P. M. (2006). Comparison of high-grade and low-grade mobilization techniques in the management of adhesive capsulitis of the shoulder: Randomized controlled trial. *Physical Therapy, 86,* 355–368.

Vlaeyen, J., Kole-Snijders, A., Boeren, R., & Van Eek, H. (1995). Fear of movement/(re)injury in chronic low back pain and its relation to behavioral performance. *Pain, 62,* 363–367.

Waddel, G., Newton, M., Henderson, I., Somerville D., & Main, C. J. (1993). A fear-avoidance beliefs questionnaire and the role of fear-avoidance beliefs in chronic low back pain and disability. *Pain, 52,* 157–168.

Wajon, A., & Ada, L. (2005). No difference between two splint and exercise regimens for people with osteoarthritis of the thumb: A randomized controlled trial. *Australian Journal of Physiotherapy, 51,* 245–249.

Waling, K., Sundelin, G., Ahlgren, C., & Jarvholm, B. (2000). Perceived pain before and after three exercise programs—A controlled clinical trial of women with work-related trapezius myalgia. *Pain, 85,* 201–207.

Ware, J. E., Snow, K. K., Kosinski, M., & Gandek B. (2000). *SF–36 Health Survey: Manual and interpretation guide.* Lincoln, RI: QualityMetric.

Warwick, L., & Seradge, H. (1995). Early versus late range of motion following cubital tunnel surgery. *Journal of Hand Therapy, 8,* 245–248.

Weinstock-Zlotnick, G., Torres-Gray, D., & Segal, R. (2004). Effect of pressure garment work gloves on hand function in patients with hand burns: A pilot study. *Journal of Hand Therapy, 17,* 368–376.

Werner, R. A., Franzblau, A., & Gell, N. (2005). Randomized controlled trial of nocturnal splinting for active workers with symptoms of carpal tunnel syndrome. *Archives of Physical Medicine and Rehabilitation, 86,* 1–7.

Wessel, J. (2004). The effectiveness of hand exercises for persons with rheumatoid arthritis: A systematic review. *Journal of Hand Therapy, 17,* 174–180.

Whaley, M. H., Brubaker, P., & Otto, R. M. (2006). *American College of Sports Medicine's guidelines for exercise testing and prescription* (7th ed.). Philadelphia: Lippincott Williams & Wilkins.

Willer, B., Ottenbacher, K. J., & Coad, M. L. (1994). The Community Integration Questionnaire: A comparative examination. *American Journal of Physical Medicine and Rehabilitation, 73,* 103–111.

Williams, R., & Myers, A. (1998). Functional Abilities Confidence Scale: A clinical measure for injured workers with acute low back pain. *Physical Therapy, 6,* 625–634.

Williams, R. M., Westmorland, M. G., Schmuck, G., & MacDermid, J. C. (2004). Effectiveness of workplace rehabilitation interventions in the treatment of work-related upper extremity disorders: A systematic review. *Journal of Hand Therapy, 17,* 267–273.

Wilson, B. A., Alderman, N., Burgess, P., Emslie, H., & Evans, J. J. (1996). *Behavioural Assessment of Dysexecutive Syndrome.* San Antonio, TX: Harcourt Assessment.

World Health Organization. (2001). *International classification of functioning, disability, and health.* Geneva, Switzerland: Author.

World Health Organization. (2003). *The burden of musculoskeletal conditions at the start of the new millennium* (WHO Technical Report Series). Geneva, Switzerland: Author.

■ ■ ■